JOYSPAN

JOYSPAN

A SHORT GUIDE TO ENJOYING YOUR LONG LIFE

Dr Kerry Burnight

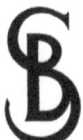

First published in Great Britain in 2025 by Short Books, an imprint of
Octopus Publishing Group Ltd
Carmelite House
50 Victoria Embankment
London EC4Y 0DZ
www.octopusbooks.co.uk

An Hachette UK Company
www.hachette.co.uk

The authorized representative in the EEA is Hachette Ireland,
8 Castlecourt Centre, Dublin 15, D15 XTP3, Ireland (email: info@hbgi.ie)

Copyright © 2025 Kerry Burnight, PhD

All rights reserved. No part of this work may be reproduced or utilized in any form or by any means, electronic or mechanical, including photocopying, recording or by any information storage and retrieval system, without the prior written permission of the publisher.

ISBN 978-1-78325-634-1
eISBN 978-1-78325-632-7

A CIP catalogue record for this book is available from the British Library.

Printed and bound in Great Britain.

1 3 5 7 9 10 8 6 4 2

This FSC® label means that materials used for the product have been responsibly sourced.

Disclaimer: This book is not intended as a substitute for medical advice of physicians. The reader should regularly consult a physician in all matters relating to his or her health, and particularly in respect of any symptoms that may require diagnosis or medical attention.

The publisher is not responsible for websites (or their content) that are not owned by the publisher.

To Betty and John Parker, who taught me to dive into life.
To my love, Todd Burnight, who swims with me through every tide.
To Beau, Claire, and Elle Burnight, who inspire us to float,
breathe, and enjoy the water.

JOYSPAN

Contents

Introduction   xi

PART I
WHY YOUR JOYSPAN MATTERS

Chapter 1. What Is Joyspan?	3
Chapter 2. How Your Joyspan Affects Your Lifespan	25
Chapter 3. How Your Joyspan Affects Your Healthspan	50

PART II
WHAT STRENGTHENS YOUR JOYSPAN

Chapter 4. Grow with Joy	75
Chapter 5. Connect to Joy	103
Chapter 6. Adapt with Joy	129
Chapter 7. Give with Joy	152

PART III
HOW TO CREATE YOUR JOYSPAN

Chapter 8. Filling Your Joytank	177
Chapter 9. When Your Joyspan Dips	199

Conclusion: The Joyspan Legacy	219
Resources	223
Notes	225
Acknowledgments	233
About the Author	235

Introduction

People ask all the time: What's Betty's secret?

Betty is my ninety-six-year-old mother. She lives on her own, is as sharp as ever, belly-laughs with friends, and never forgets a birthday or condolence card. Family, neighbors—even strangers—can't get enough of her.

But here's the thing—Betty has never been particularly athletic, enjoys dessert, sips the occasional cocktail, and is the first to admit she didn't always have the best attitude when she was younger. So how is she thriving in her later years?

Spoiler alert: It's not her genes and it's not just luck.

Her secret isn't perfect health or a life free from hardship. In fact, it's not a secret at all—it's science.

As a gerontologist, I've spent decades researching the factors that enable people to thrive in the second half of life. In this book, I share the proven strategies that have helped Betty maximize well-being in longevity—and that will help you do the same.

When we talk about longevity, we often focus on lifespan—how long we live—or healthspan—how many of those years are in good health. But what's the point of a long, healthy life if you're not enjoying it?

That's where joyspan comes in—the key to a fulfilling long life. It's about more than just physical health; it's about cultivating internal strength—the ability to grow, connect, adapt, and give, all life long.

We are all aging. Whether you're twenty-three or a hundred and three, the best time to invest in your joyspan is right now.

Let's get started.

A NEW WAY TO LOOK AT AGE

Anyone who says, "Age is just a number," has not reached the high numbers. Aging is not easy, and "forever young" is not a plan. Regardless of how many burpees you can do or protein smoothies you chug, the passing of time brings challenges. Roles that you relished change, words on the menus seem to shrink, necks sag, diagnoses arise.

On the other hand, aging is not the downhill slide that people believe it is. A multibillion-dollar antiaging industry profits when you feel awful about yourself and fear aging like the plague. The tragedy of aging is not that we will all grow old and die, but that aging has been made unnecessarily, and at times excruciatingly, painful and humiliating. Aging does not have to be this way. When it comes to longevity, the primary focus has been upon lifespan, the length of life.

More recently, the scope has expanded beyond years of life to *years of life in good health*, or healthspan. This is a welcomed shift, because we all want to live as healthy as possible for as long as possible.

But there's a catch. A long life, even a long life in good health, doesn't mean much if you don't like your life. As geriatrician Dr. Louise Aronson observes, "We've added a couple of decades, essentially an entire generation, onto our lives, and we haven't figured out how to handle that."[1]

What we've been missing is a practical vocabulary and approach to maximizing the quality of our long lives. We need a science-based, how-to guide for creating long lives characterized by inner well-being. It's not enough to have a long lifespan and healthspan; we want what I call a long *joyspan*.

WHAT IS JOYSPAN?

Joyspan is the experience of well-being and satisfaction in longevity. Because the focus is upon well-being, I tried out the term "wellspan" with my patients. After more than a few people thought I was saying, "wealthspan," I started calling it "joyspan"—it's been a perfect fit. The American Psychological Association defines *joy* as the feeling that arises from a sense of well-being or satisfaction. Experiencing joy is different from feeling happy. Happiness comes and goes and is often dependent on external circumstances. Joy can be experienced even in adverse situations. More akin to contentment than to ecstasy, joy may show up in the form of a smile, but many times it does not. You cannot always ascertain someone's joy by observing them. One older woman looking at the trees through her window may be lonely and miserable, while a different older woman looking at the same trees may be experiencing great joy.

My mother, Betty, is enjoying a long joyspan. She practices what I preach: a research-based, proven approach to maximize well-being in longevity. Joyspan requires knowledge, intention, and effort and is achievable regardless of where you are starting out today. Your current approach to longevity is no doubt incomplete. In everyday media we are inundated with advice on maximizing physical fitness, but very little on how to maximize internal fitness and emotional well-being. Joyspan brings to light the robust research findings on psychological well-being, which are too often tucked away in academic journals. This book is what you need but have been missing.

To thrive in old age means to live a fulfilling, purposeful, and satisfying life despite the challenges that accompany aging. It involves maximizing physical health, cognitive function, emotional well-being, social connections, and a sense of meaning. Thriving doesn't mean being free of all health problems or challenges; rather, it emphasizes resilience, adaptability, and the ability to find joy and value in life. People don't thrive in longevity by mistake or luck. People who thrive in longevity actively maximize the quality of their lives. But how? What does the research say about HOW to thrive in life's second half? As a gerontologist, I scoured the findings of thirty-five years of empirical testing on psychological well-being in longevity. The research was conducted by experts from around the globe and points to hundreds of predictors. But the deeper I dug into the findings, the more I recognized a profound underlying pattern. The hundreds of predictors found in thousands of studies on what is necessary to thrive in longevity consistently group into four essential elements. The research showed that people with long joyspans actively commit to four critical actions:

- Grow: They continue to explore and expand.
- Connect: They put time into new and existing relationships.
- Adapt: They adjust to changing and challenging situations.
- Give: They share themselves.

Each of these elements is nonnegotiable for well-being in longevity, and you can improve in each area. Joyspan matters because without it, a long life is a drag.

MY PATH TO JOYSPAN

When I completed my PhD thirty years ago, I was in the oxymoronic position of being the youngest doctor of gerontology in the country. To me it made perfect sense—in fact, it felt like I was born a gerontologist. To start out, I came as a surprise to my middle-aged parents and my siblings, who were high school age. I was the only four-year-old in preschool whose sister was married. When kids made fun of old people, it felt personal to me. Sometimes I'd ride out the jabs in silence; other times I'd stand up for my people: the gray, the wrinkled, and the fabulous.

I taught geriatric medicine and gerontology for nineteen years at the University of California, Irvine School of Medicine. At UCI's Senior Health Center, I had a front-row seat to observe people, and their families, navigate old age. What struck me most was the radical differences in how people experienced their own aging process. For some, it is a frustrating, degrading, painful trajectory of ever-increasing decline. For others, there is visible delight, spirituality, and joy in occupying their eighth, ninth, and tenth decades.

The vast majority of my career has focused upon the former group, those suffering in old age. What I've seen has burned my eyes and left scars on my heart. Blue-eyed Mrs. C., who endured searing physical pain and profound loneliness. Proud Mr. R., who had to choose between needed medication and a meal. Miss T., who cared lovingly for her brother with Down syndrome until she developed Alzheimer's disease, and the two were found in conditions that haunt me to this day.

Dr. Laura Mosqueda is my mentor, friend, and a gifted geriatrician. She and I had the privilege of creating and codirecting the nation's first Elder Abuse Forensic Center, which investigates cases of elder abuse. What we learned from thousands of cases of elder abuse and neglect is that no one is immune to finding themselves in dire situations in old age.

We learned that loneliness kills, and that isolation is a key risk factor. We came to understand that neglect and mistreatment don't occur just in dilapidated shacks, but also behind the closed doors of beautiful homes. Suffering in old age is not a "they" problem; it's an "us" problem. We found that after the abuse, neglect, or financial exploitation occurs, it is the older adult who feels shame instead of the perpetrator—which is heartbreaking and infuriating. Other times, there is no one at fault, only an awful no-win situation with suffering all around.

Many days I drove home from work in tears, my blouse doubling as a tissue. Laura and I received the National Crime Victims' Service Award from the US attorney general, and though I should have been proud, I remember feeling awful on the flight home. I had an image of myself sitting at the base of a skateboard ramp. I was doing my best to bandage up people when they hit the elder abuse pavement at the end of the ramp, but scars and suffering remained. I realized that the real goal was to get to the top of that skateboard ramp and provide people with the equipment they needed for the experiences of later life.

The purpose of this book is to fortify you and those you love for these unprecedented long lives. I want you to thrive during your entire life.

ABOUT THIS BOOK

I've divided *Joyspan* into three sections.

Part 1 explains why your joyspan matters. Chapter 1 defines joyspan and highlights joyspanners who have preceded you. Chapters 2 and 3 delve into how joyspan affects your lifespan and healthspan.

Part 2 explains what you need to do to strengthen your joyspan. Chapter 4 is a deep dive into the first essential element of joyspan, lifelong growth. Chapter 5 provides practical information on how to create and strengthen your community and connection in the second half of life. In chapter 6 you will learn how adaptability contributes to joyspan and how to maximize your adaptability. Chapter 7 shows how giving back unlocks your life purpose and provides meaning.

Part 3 reveals how to create your joyspan for a life you will enjoy living all the way to the end. Chapter 8 shows you how to fill your joytank, while chapter 9 gives you the tools you'll need when your joyspan dips. I examine common struggles such as feeling like a burden, mobility and health obstacles, and loss.

Within each of the three parts, you'll see recurring elements. *Joyspanners* are mini-profiles of adults embodying the elements of joyspan. *Joy Practices* offer activities and exercises to go deeper into your exploration of what creates a long joyspan. Finally, *Joyspan Matrices* are examples of how real people are applying the four elements of joyspan.

I've been thinking about old age for a long time. Thirty-three years ago, I wrote this poem in response to my English professor's prompt: "What do you care about?" What I cared about, what I still care about, was older people. The poem, called "We Are They," ends this way:

Yet somehow, we row closer still, toward the mighty river's end.
The moans they are among us now, at last we understand.

We are they, and we can make choices now, here in gentler tides, while we are miles up the river.

What I want you to gain from reading this book is hope. A good and joyful second half of life is an inside job. Just as the physical self is made up of cells, the inner self is made up of thoughts. According to the National Research Foundation, humans have around sixty thousand thoughts per day. Like cells, thoughts are often small and seemingly innocuous. Taken together, however, thoughts become the inner self. As we grow older, we can't hide behind a fresh face or body. The inner self takes center stage, and it can be glorious. I know because I've seen the radiance of joyspan in thousands of older adults. I want that for you.

PART I

Why Your Joyspan Matters

CHAPTER 1

What Is Joyspan?

I had two grandmothers, Eda and Charlotte.

"Don't ever get old, Kerry," Gram Eda told me. She was only sixty-four. "Back in the day, I was actually useful." Eda believed that growing older was all downhill, and she made her decisions based upon that belief.

Eda stopped cultivating relationships with family and friends. Visits consisted of us sitting around staring at her while she talked about her unfair life, saying, "I got a bad break, losing Theodore, and then becoming crippled with this damn arthritis." I could hardly wait until it was time to leave our visits.

Eda could not accept the older version of herself. She had a lot to give but couldn't see it. For example, I longed to have her take an interest in me and to tell me about her younger self. Her stories were left untold, and memories were never created. Eda *believed* older would be awful, and she was right. Although she lived eighty-one years, her joyspan was less than sixty years.

My maternal grandmother, Charlotte, held a very different view of aging. Like Eda, Charlotte lived alone on a small, fixed income after her husband's passing. She saw aging as the opportunity to do more living. "Kerry," she said one day, "you may join me on my walk tomorrow, but I leave right at seven a.m. Be ready to go or I'll go without you." I was ready. The walk took us to a hidden greenbelt covered with tiny grazing bunnies. She exposed me to the fresh quiet of morning, a world I usually slept through.

Charlotte made it a point to get outside every day. She was equally committed to continued intellectual growth. She took notes when she watched the news. "I like to know which leaders are from which countries, and what they are doing," she'd explain. My mom saved these TV notes—the names Pierre Trudeau (Canada) and Isabel Perón (the first woman president of a world country, Argentina) scrawled in her curly penmanship. As Charlotte's longtime friends began to predecease her, she created a women's reading group to discuss books, share meals, and listen to music. Charlotte only had one child, my mother, Betty, yet she was rich with family. She often telephoned Betty, her three grandchildren, their spouses, and her eleven great-grandchildren. When she could no longer walk unassisted, Charlotte adapted her daily workouts to her walker. In her late eighties, Charlotte grew frail, but she always saw her value, always knew she had something to give. The focused attention and encouragement she gave me impacted the trajectory of my life. Charlotte *believed* being older would be just fine, and she was right. Her joyspan was as long as her lifespan—eighty-nine years.

We remember Charlotte with fondness, and Eda with sorrow. How do you wish to be remembered? What specifically enables some people to thrive in longevity while others languish? The attention they give to cultivating their joyspan.

INTRODUCING JOYSPAN

Joyspan is the experience of psychological well-being and satisfaction in longevity. It is the response to the question: *Why* do you want to live longer? For what? For whom?

In a world obsessed with living longer, Joyspan is about living better.

We've been missing a practical vocabulary and approach to maximizing the *quality* of our long lives. Joyspan is a science-based "how-to" for creating a long life characterized by inner well-being. The goal is to live as long as possible with as much quality of life as possible.

> Longevity is not just a number of years (lifespan).
> It's not even the number of years lived in good health (healthspan).
> It's how many years you enjoy living (joyspan).

How do years of life intersect with quality of life? Let's think about it with a simple diagram. The "Years of Life" axis is divided into two categories: long life and short life; and the "Quality of Life" axis is divided into two categories: high well-being and low well-being. The resulting four quadrants are summarized in figure 1.

FIGURE 1. The Length and Quality of Your Life

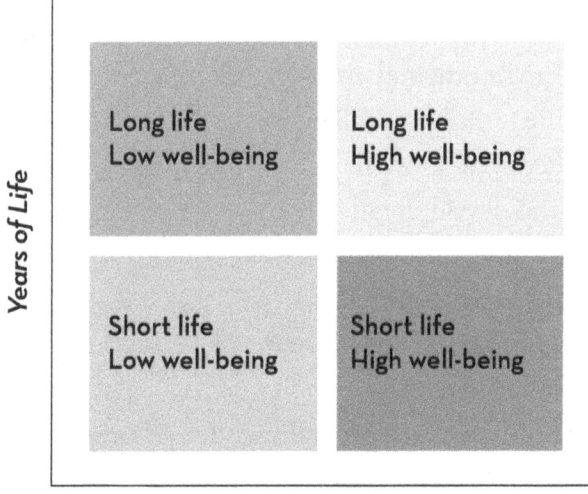

Because we are interested in longevity, let's focus on the upper squares of the quadrant, representing people with long lives. There are two options: (1) the upper left quadrant: a long life with low well-being; and (2) the upper right quadrant: a long life with high well-being. In other words, suffering or joyspan. That's an easy one; you opt for the upper right quadant, all day, every day. You opt for joyspan.

But how? What are the predictors of joyspan according to the research? Thousands of studies in the fields of gerontology, psychology, sociology, neuroscience, biology, epigenetics, and philosophy have posed this question.

In her seminal 1989 paper, "Happiness Is Everything, or Is It?," Dr. Carol Ryff laid the foundation for the Psychological Well-Being model (PWB model), offering a multidimensional perspective on what it means to live well beyond mere pleasure-seeking.[1] The PWB model was influenced by existential, humanistic, and developmental psychology—particularly the work of Carl Jung, Erik Erikson, Abraham Maslow, and Viktor Frankl. The PWB model identifies six core components that predict positive functioning throughout life:

1. Autonomy: The ability to make independent choices and resist social pressures.
2. Environmental mastery: Competence in managing everyday life tasks and challenges.
3. Personal growth: A continued openness to new experiences and development.
4. Positive relationships with others: Developing deep, meaningful social connections.
5. Purpose in life: A sense of direction, meaning, and future-oriented goals.
6. Self-acceptance: A realistic view of oneself, acknowledging both strengths and weaknesses.

The Psychological Well-Being model has been tested extensively in projects such as the MIDUS (Midlife in the United States) survey and the Survey of Midlife Development in Japan. These studies focus on how well-being evolves across the course of a life, exploring the roles of life transitions, social roles, and health changes. Findings confirm that even as physical health declines with age, many older adults report high levels of personal growth, purpose, and self-acceptance, suggesting resilience in psychological well-being. This finding holds true in studies in other countries as well. For example, the international Survey of Midlife Development found that cultural differences shaped certain aspects of well-being (for example, autonomy), but purpose, relationships, and self-acceptance remained important across all contexts.[2]

Taken together, thousands of studies from around the world confirm that psychological well-being is dynamic, meaning that it can be changed, and it can be maintained or even enhanced with age, especially when individuals stay engaged, maintain social connections, and find new sources of meaning.

The joyspan model builds on the foundation of the Psychological Well-Being model, with an additional element shown to predict well-being in later life: adaptability. Developed by Israeli researcher Dr. Hod Orkibi, the creative adaptability framework is the capacity to generate cognitive, emotional, and behavioral responses to changing and stressful situations.[3] His research reveals the power of adaptability in older adults to foster psychological flexibility and well-being in later life. As we grow older, adaptability helps us manage transitions like retirement or health challenges through proactive engagement and emotional regulation. Findings reveal that older adults with higher adaptability skills experience greater resilience and personal growth.

——— JOY PRACTICE: ———
The Joyspan Inventory

How is your joyspan? Take the Joyspan Inventory by circling your answers to the eight questions below. Be as honest as possible—this is just your baseline. You can improve it!

GROW

1. For me, life has been a continuous process of learning, changing, and growth.

Strongly agree	Somewhat agree	Slightly agree	Neither agree nor disagree	Slightly disagree	Somewhat disagree	Strongly disagree
7	6	5	4	3	2	1

2. I think it is important to have new experiences that challenge how I think about myself and the world.

Strongly agree	Somewhat agree	Slightly agree	Neither agree nor disagree	Slightly disagree	Somewhat disagree	Strongly disagree
7	6	5	4	3	2	1

CONNECT

3. I have experienced many warm and trusting relationships with others.

Strongly agree	Somewhat agree	Slightly agree	Neither agree nor disagree	Slightly disagree	Somewhat disagree	Strongly disagree
7	6	5	4	3	2	1

4. I enjoy mutual conversations with family members and friends.

Strongly agree	Somewhat agree	Slightly agree	Neither agree nor disagree	Slightly disagree	Somewhat disagree	Strongly disagree
7	6	5	4	3	2	1

ADAPT

5. I try to think about stress from a new perspective.

Strongly agree	Somewhat agree	Slightly agree	Neither agree nor disagree	Slightly disagree	Somewhat disagree	Strongly disagree
7	6	5	4	3	2	1

6. I adopt new behaviors to help me through changed circumstances.

Strongly agree	Somewhat agree	Slightly agree	Neither agree nor disagree	Slightly disagree	Somewhat disagree	Strongly disagree
7	6	5	4	3	2	1

GIVE

7. People would describe me as a giving person, willing to share my time with others.

Strongly agree	Somewhat agree	Slightly agree	Neither agree nor disagree	Slightly disagree	Somewhat disagree	Strongly disagree
7	6	5	4	3	2	1

8. I have a sense of direction and purpose in my life.

Strongly agree	Somewhat agree	Slightly agree	Neither agree nor disagree	Slightly disagree	Somewhat disagree	Strongly disagree
7	6	5	4	3	2	1

To score, add up the numbers of the answers you circled.

GROW = _____

CONNECT = _____

ADAPT = _____

GIVE = _____

The higher the score, the better. Take note of your lowest and highest scores. See if they change over time.

THE JOYSPAN MATRIX

The Joyspan Matrix is how you take action. The definition of a matrix is an environment in which the elements of something develop. The Joyspan Matrix is the environment in which the four elements of joyspan develop. The Joyspan Matrix consists of the four essential actions: Grow, Connect, Adapt, and Give. As depicted below, each of the four elements is based on research into the topics shown in figure 2.

FIGURE 2. Four Actions Associated with Thriving in Longevity

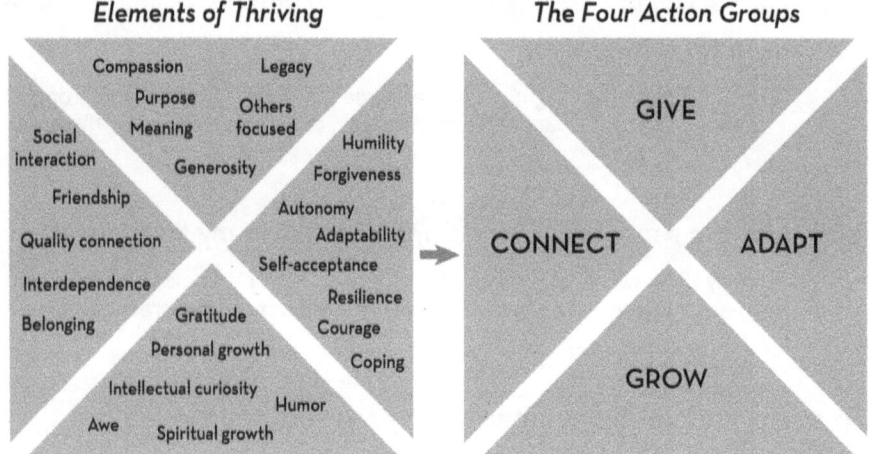

The Four Actions Groups of Thriving

For example, the element *Connect* is drawn from the research showing the importance of social interaction, friendship, quality relationships, belonging, and interdependence. Each of the elements is captured in an action word to highlight your active role in maximizing your joyspan (see figure 3).

Each of the elements is essential to Joyspan and each can be improved—even radically improved.

GROW is your determination to continue developing as a person.
CONNECT is your dedication to building relationships with other people.
ADAPT is your desire and ability to adjust to life's inevitable challenges.
GIVE is your willingness to share yourself to enrich the lives of others.

FIGURE 3. The Joyspan Matrix

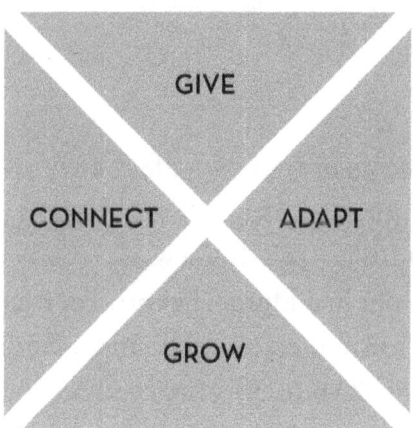

Like physical fitness, your emotional and psychological fitness—your joyspan—takes daily attention and effort. Figure 4 is a joyspan matrix in action from the life of my friend Joe. Like everyone, Joe's joyspan matrix is dynamic and always changing. This was Joe's matrix two years after the death of his wife, Laura.

You will find additional real-life examples of the Joyspan Matrix in action below. As you read through these real-life examples and then go on about your life, you'll start to become aware of these four

FIGURE 4. Joyspan Matrix in Action: Joe, Age 78

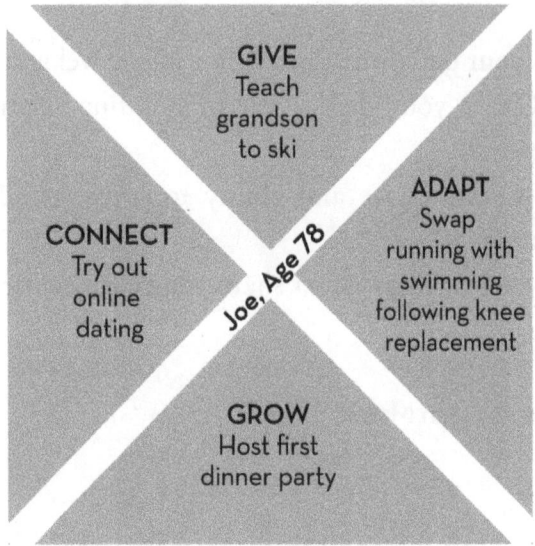

critical action elements in your own life. Often, you will find yourself strong and active in some elements and lagging in other elements. That's normal, and with this framework, you'll be able to identify where you need to put in additional effort. For example, you may find yourself actively growing, connecting, and adapting, but realize you aren't actively giving of yourself. When you become aware of this, you will be able to take more action in giving and watch your joy rise.

WHAT IS JOY?

Joy is the experience of contentment, gratitude, and meaning, regardless of our external circumstance. Joy is not simply feeling happy. Joy encompasses quality of life and the ability to contribute to the world with a sense of meaning and purpose. Archbishop Desmond Tutu explained, "While happiness is often seen as being dependent on external circumstances, joy is not." Joy, by definition, cannot be the goal. "If you...say 'I want joy,' clenching your teeth with determination," advises the Dalai Lama, "this is the quickest way of missing the joy bus."[4]

> "Joy does not simply happen to us. We have to choose joy and keep choosing it every day."
> —Henri Nouwen, Dutch Catholic priest, professor, and writer

The concept of joy has ancient roots, with some of the earliest references to it found in religious texts, philosophical writings, and poetry. In the Sumerian text *The Epic of Gilgamesh* (2100 BC), passages describe moments of joy through friendship and celebration and mark one of humanity's earliest reflections on interpersonal joy. *The Rigveda* (1500–1200 BC), part of the Indian Vedas, includes hymns that celebrate joy, bliss, and gratitude toward the divine. Concepts like *ānanda* (bliss and joy) are central to both spiritual fulfillment and cosmic harmony. In the Hebrew Bible (1000 BC), joy is seen as a gift from God, connected to faith, worship, and righteousness. Psalm 16:11 states: "You make known to me the path of life; in your presence there is fullness of joy."[5] The *Tao Te Ching* by Laozi (sixth century BC) suggests that simplicity and contentment lead to joy. The work advocates for a peaceful life, removed from excess and ambition. The teachings of the Buddha (fifth–fourth century BC) emphasize joy (*pīti* in the Pali language) as a mental quality associated with spiritual practice. The joy from meditation and insight is considered integral to achieving enlightenment.

All these ancient texts, along with millions of writings on joy created since then, highlight different forms of joy—whether through divine connection, human relationships, or inner peace—and reflect how joy has been regarded as an essential part of life for millennia.

> "Live in joy, in love, even among those who hate. Live in joy, in health, even among the afflicted. Live in joy, in peace, even among the troubled."
> —*Dhammapāla*

If we look through the prisms of neuroscience, philosophy, psychology, sociology, and evolution, we find additional ways to think about joy. Neuroscientists, for example, have demonstrated how joy activates key areas in the brain, which impacts behavior and emotional well-being. A part of the brain called the nucleus accumbens plays a vital role in experiencing joy, which in turn impacts neurotransmitters associated with pleasure and reward. Joy is linked to the release of both dopamine and serotonin. Specifically, dopamine surges in this region during positive experiences, reinforcing behaviors that lead to joy and motivate individuals to seek similar rewarding activities in the future. Functional MRI studies reveal that joy activates regions such as the prefrontal cortex and the amygdala, two parts of the brain that govern emotions and positive experiences.[6]

From a philosophical perspective, thinkers like Aristotle considered joy to be part of eudaimonia (a meaningful, flourishing life), connected with virtues rather than fleeting pleasure. In existential philosophy, joy is associated with moments of authenticity and transcendence in which individuals feel fully aligned with themselves or life's purpose (e.g., Kierkegaard's work on joy rooted in faith).

In a branch of psychology called positive psychology, joy contributes to mental thriving, and studies show that joy enhances resilience and social bonds. Theorist Barbara Fredrickson suggests that joy can broaden thought processes and encourage creative exploration. [7]

From a sociological vantage point, joy can be communal, as seen in celebrations or rituals where individuals feel uplifted by shared experiences (e.g., festivals and sports events). Different cultures value and express joy uniquely. For example, "joie de vivre" in French culture emphasizes savoring life's pleasures, while some Eastern cultures associate joy with contentment and harmony. In evolutionary science, joy is shown to encourage social bonding and cooperative behavior, which are essential for survival and community building. Children exhibit spontaneous joy, often tied to play and exploration, which fosters cognitive and emotional growth.

JOY IN SPIRITUALITY

Joy in spirituality is described as a deep, transcendent experience that arises from connection—with God, nature, art, and meaningful human interactions—beyond the fulfillment of personal desires. Joy reflects a sense of unity, presence, and peace, often cultivated through mindful engagement with the seen and the unseen parts of life. For example, nature instills a sense of joy and wonder by reconnecting us with the rhythms of the earth. As John Muir beautifully remarked: "In every walk with nature, one receives far more than he seeks." Joy is not just about individual gain but about aligning with something larger than oneself.

Loving interactions, when meaningful and authentic, elicit joy that transcends personal desires. I first typed the sentence as "loving human interactions" but then our dogs walked up to me, and after a big hug, I corrected the sentence. Sociologist Brené Brown, in her research, emphasizes that joy arises from vulnerability and authenticity in relationships.[8] Joy is found in moments of shared love—whether in community, friendship, or small acts of kindness.

Art has long been seen as a source of transcendent joy, capable of stirring emotions and connecting individuals to deeper meanings. Philosopher Friedrich von Schiller suggested that engaging with beauty through art fosters an elevated state of joy, liberating the mind and soul from mundane concerns. Consider his work "Ode to Joy," which inspired Beethoven's Ninth Symphony—a testament to how artistic beauty can elicit collective joy and shared human experience.

> **"Joy collected over time fuels resilience—ensuring we'll have reservoirs of emotional strength when hard things do happen."**
> —*Brené Brown, researcher and writer*

Both religious and secular spirituality emphasize mindfulness—the practice of being fully present in the moment—as a path to joy. Philosopher Alan Watts suggested that joy is inherent in the experience of living fully in the present, unburdened by regrets or worries about the future. He explains that the real secret of life is to be completely engaged with what you are doing in the here and now. He advises that instead of calling it work, we can realize it is play.[9] Mindfulness in daily activities opens the door to simple, everyday joys, reinforcing the idea that joy is accessible when we are fully present.

Secular spirituality points to the profound fulfillment of cultivating joy that goes beyond material or self-centered pursuits.

Joy matters. Joy is a profound emotional experience that transcends circumstances, enhancing well-being, personal growth, and social connection. Joy bridges internal fulfillment with external engagement, whether through personal achievements, spirituality, or shared moments of celebration. Joy matters all life long and is especially important in later years when we experience more challenges.

Now that you have a broad understanding of joy, how do you apply it to your joyspan? Let's start with your mindset.

HOW THE TWO AGING MINDSETS IMPACT JOYSPAN

Regardless of your current age, you hold one of two mindsets: aging as decline or aging as continued growth.

The decline mindset believes everything gets worse as you grow older and then you die. Sadly, this mindset is the most prevalent. From the time we were toddlers we've been fed a steady diet of "Old is bad" messaging. Remember Hansel and Gretel? The story teaches us that old women are ugly witches who will boil and eat you. The impact of negative attitudes on aging is staggering. The World Health Organization (WHO) estimates that 6.3 million cases of depression worldwide can be attributed to the effects of ageism. Internalized ageism is a risk factor for depression, anxiety, and suicidal ideation.[10]

Research shows that people can alter their largely unrecognized assumptions about growing older and assume more control over them. Those who expect lifelong growth fare better than those who expect aging to be all decline. More than four hundred scientific studies have demonstrated the impact of individuals' beliefs about aging. Dr. Becca Levy and her team at Yale University have proved that those with positive beliefs about aging lived seven and a half years longer than those who held negative beliefs about aging! And it's not just the length of our lives but the quality that is impacted by our beliefs. Dr. Levy found that people with positive age beliefs maintained better physical and functional health over an eighteen-year period.[11]

The growth mindset sees aging as a time of continued progress in becoming who you are. This mindset recognizes not only the challenges and losses of growing older but also the opportunities and strengths.

Take my neighbor Dee, who is eighty-one. A few days ago, I saw her on her front porch while I was walking the dogs, and she waved me over so she could tell me all about her sore hands, the "absolute drivel" on TV, and how bad the hot weather makes her feel. Because Dee sees her life as a downward free fall, she's stopped showing up for it. She does not pursue her former interests, reach out to friends, or challenge herself. Why bother? If you believe there is nothing you can do to impact your life as you grow older, it makes sense to stop putting in the effort. The long hours spent in her recliner have seriously weakened her legs, which she blames on the curse of being old. Our conversations never have room for topics beyond her discomfort. Despite our many conversations, Dee doesn't know anything about me other than the fact that I have two golden retrievers. There isn't any space for me to share my life, because her life, as miserable as she finds it, is the topic that dominates her mind. Dee definitely holds a decline mindset.

I often run into another neighbor, Joan, who walks the same loop I do. I absolutely love it when I run into Joan. She is eighty-two and just radiant. Soon after our middle daughter was diagnosed with a brain tumor, I saw Joan and she noticed right away that something was off. She asked me what was going on in a way that felt safe for me to share. She listened intensely, then suggested ways to adjust to this "new normal." Joan has had so many new normals. Always very interested in something—a new plant she's potted, a new recipe, an interesting book, an upcoming art exhibit—Joan has a growth mindset. Growing older is about, well, growing, about becoming. Joan knows that interior strengths can continue to develop throughout life. I once told Joan how much I admire her attitude, and she laughed, saying, "I find life fascinating. I'm still growing now, just as I have in every other phase of my life."

The chart below summarizes how the two aging mindsets impact, either negatively or positively, your joyspan.

	Decline Mindset	Growth Mindset
Aging Expectations	Growing older results in decline in every area of life.	Growing older results in decline in some areas and improvement in other areas.
Perspective on Control	The quality of my life is out of my control.	The quality of my life is up to me.
Level of Effort	Minimal—why bother when effort is fruitless?	Effort can improve quality of life.
Reaction to Obstacles	Gives up in the face of challenge.	Persists in the face of challenge.
Relationships	How can you help me?	How can I help you?

Could Dee move from a decline mindset to a growth mindset? Yes. I have seen the benefits of the mindset shift in action. Moving to a growth mindset improves, and very literally saves, lives. But given the power of antiaging messaging, a decline mindset path is far more commonly traveled. Most people don't know there is a choice, so they head in this direction by default. With a decline mindset, you see yourself as less valuable and less capable and so others believe that is true of you. Health challenges reinforce your belief that it is all downhill. The passing of loved ones further confirms that age is stacked against you.

In contrast, on the growth mindset path, people capitalize on what they do better as they age. Those traveling this way are not clinging to youth but decisively striding toward learning and development. They proactively challenge the belief that growing older inevitably leads to decline in all facets of life. Instead, the continued growth path focuses on the opportunities and improvements that come with experience and maturity.

——— JOY PRACTICE: ———
What's Your Aging Mindset?

Answer these four questions to see if you lean toward a **growth mindset** or a **decline mindset** around aging. For each question, choose the option that best reflects your belief.

How do you view getting older?

    a. An opportunity for continued growth and expansion.
    b. A time of physical, mental, and social decline.

How do you approach challenges that come with aging (setbacks or health issues)?

    a. They are a normal part of growth and are just new obstacles to work around or adapt to.
    b. Setbacks and challenges are signs that I am slowing down and losing capability.

What role do social connections play for you as you age?

    a. It's essential to stay connected and meet new people.
    b. It's natural for social life to shrink with age.

What is your attitude toward physical activity?

    a. Staying active is key to maintaining health and joy.
    b. Exercise becomes too hard or less important as you get older.

RESULTS

MOSTLY "a." ANSWERS:

You have a **growth mindset** around aging! You view getting older as an opportunity to continue learning, adapting, and connecting with others. You believe that aging is just another stage for personal growth and fulfillment.

Mostly "b." answers:

You lean toward a **decline mindset** around aging. You may see aging as a time of loss and reduced capacity. Recognizing this mindset can be a first step toward shifting to a more positive view of aging, focusing on the opportunities still available.

Shifting from a decline mindset to a growth mindset involves intentional changes in both attitudes and actions. Awareness is the first step—catch yourself in the act of saying, thinking, or hearing negative comments about aging, such as *I'm too old to learn that; I can't wear that; I'm having a senior moment.* You'll be surprised how many anti-aging comments you'll hear in your own head. Next, proactively replace the negative and self-limiting beliefs with empowering assertions of what is possible. Instead of dwelling on what you can no longer do, shift your attention to what you *can* do. This mindset strengthens resilience.

Practice gratitude, which reshapes your internal dialogue and helps you adopt a more accurate, more optimistic view of aging. Get out there and engage in mentoring, creative projects, or paid or volunteer work. Remind yourself of what you *can* do to improve lives, and do it. Hang out with positive influences—people who inspire a proactive approach to making the most of their long lives.

YOU CAN HAVE A GREAT JOYSPAN NO MATTER WHERE YOU ARE NOW

Longevity is determined by your genetics. Right? Wrong.

It's easy to feel limited by family history, but research shows that what we do every day—exercise, meaningful connections, healthy eating, and stress management—outweighs genetic predispositions. For instance, people with genetic risks for diseases like heart issues or dementia can delay or even avoid them with proper habits.

That's because genetics influences only about 25 percent of how long we live, while *lifestyle choices* determine a whopping 75 percent.[12] This means your daily actions and decisions hold incredible power in shaping not just your lifespan but also the quality of those years. Choosing to remain active, engaged, and optimistic plays a critical role in fostering longevity and mental well-being.

> "Your habits have more power to shape your health than your genes ever will."
> —Kerry Burnight, gerontologist and self-quoter

We are not passive participants in the aging process. Each choice can build resilience, adaptability, and purpose—qualities that extend life and add vitality. Instead of focusing on what genetics might limit, embrace the power of your actions. Aging with a growth mindset isn't just about avoiding decline—it's about continuing to thrive by exploring, learning, connecting, and giving back. The path to longevity lies not in hoping for good genes but in nurturing your body and mind through each phase of life. With small but meaningful shifts, you can shape the future you want, no matter your starting point.

At fifty-nine, Cindy was in a rut. She had thrived in her career as a physiotherapist raised five successful sons, and enjoyed an active lifestyle. But now that her children were grown and her career had slowed, she felt purposeless, like her energy was fading, that her looks were no longer a source of confidence. Cindy wondered, "Who am I now, and what's the use, anyway?"

Her turning point came during a conversation with her great-aunt

Eloise, who was then eighty-nine. Eloise told her, "You've spent years investing in others. What would happen if you invested in yourself? Could you start with one simple change?"

Unconvinced but wanting to satisfy her aunt, Cindy began exploring activities she thought might be fulfilling or even fun. She signed up for a photography class, using her camera to capture beauty in ways she hadn't noticed before. She joined a yoga group, not to excel but to nurture her body, and discovered joy in flexibility and mindfulness.

Cindy also reconnected with her community by mentoring young physiotherapists. Helping others reignited her sense of purpose, and every new connection built her confidence. Over time, she embraced her evolving self—not as a diminished version of who she *was*, but as someone constantly growing into *the best version of herself*. Now in her eighties, Cindy reflects on her journey with pride. "Life is a series of chapters," she says. "The story doesn't stop—it just gets richer." Her story shows that fulfillment isn't about clinging to the past but embracing the opportunities in every stage of life. Cindy's choice to shift her mindset transformed her future, and she is enjoying a long joyspan.

Now that you understand why your joyspan matters, in the next few chapters we'll see how it matters to your lifespan and your healthspan.

JOYSPANNER: Dick Van Dyke

Dick Van Dyke is an American actor, comedian, singer, and dancer whose career has spanned more than seven decades. Born on December 13, 1925, in West Plains, Missouri, Van Dyke became a household name through his versatility and charm, leaving an indelible mark on television, film, and stage.

Here are some examples of why and how he had a very long joyspan.

GROW: Showcasing his continued growth, Van Dyke at age ninety-one performed in *Mary Poppins Returns* (2018). "It lit me up," he says. "I still danced on a table, just much more carefully this time."

CONNECT: Van Dyke maintains close relationships with his four children as well as his "friends from work," such as Julie Andrews. He married his second wife, Arlene Silver, at age eighty-seven.

ADAPT: Throughout his life, Van Dyke has been open about challenges, including struggles with alcohol addiction and mental health. His 2011 autobiography, *My Lucky Life In and Out of Show Business*, reflects both resilience and gratitude. He emphasizes how laughter, dance, and a sense of play help keep him going.

GIVE: Van Dyke's a cappella group, the Vantastix, performs frequently at benefits to raise funds for children's programs and community initiatives to address homelessness.

CHAPTER 2

How Your Joyspan Affects Your Lifespan

Meet identical twins Josephine and Janice. Genetically they are exactly the same, sharing 100 percent of their DNA. Josephine lived to be ninety-seven and, up until the very end, worked part-time in a hospital gift shop and drove her 1995 white Oldsmobile to meetings of her four bridge groups, to church, and to the grocery store. Janice lived to be seventy-eight and, unlike her sister, suffered chronic medical conditions and dementia that severely curtailed her activities. Why did these genetically identical twins age so differently and have such different lifespans? How much of our lifespan is dictated by our genes?

"Lifespans are not like height, a trait that is strongly inherited," said Dr. James Vaupel, former director of the Laboratory of Survival and Longevity at the Max Planck Institute for Demographic Research. "How tall your parents are explains 80 to 90 percent of how tall you will be. But only 3 percent of how long you will live can be explained by how long your parents lived." Contrary to popular opinion, your genes are not destiny. Like Josephine and Janice, identical twins die at different times—on average, more than ten years apart.[1]

Research on thousands of twin pairs like Josephine and Janice reveals that around 25 percent of the variation in lifespan can be attributed to genetic factors. This estimate—approximately 26 percent for men and 23 percent for women—has been confirmed by multiple studies. Even more compelling, analysis of millions of family trees, derived from eighty-six million public genealogy profiles, puts the heritability of lifespan closer to 16 percent.[2] The evidence suggests that while genetics contributes to longevity, it accounts for only a fraction of the outcome. Twin studies, family history research, and genealogy analyses converge to form a striking conclusion: Lifestyle and environmental factors play a more significant role than inherited genes. This underscores the importance of cultivating emotional well-being, adopting healthy habits, and maintaining social connections to maximize the years we have.

Lifespan is not a matter of good fortune in the genetic lottery. Instead, it is shaped by the choices we make every day—how we move, the relationships we nurture, and how we care for our mental and emotional health. This finding—empowering individuals to influence their aging journey—lies at the heart of joyspan.

How long you'll live is determined by a complex mix of factors: genetic predispositions, disease, nutrition, your mother's health during pregnancy, diet, exercise, stress levels, temperament, social connection, substance abuse, subtle injuries and accidents, and simply chance events, like an auto accident or a randomly occurring mutation in a cell gene that ultimately leads to cancer. While we cannot change the genes we inherit or predict accidents, we have a profound opportunity to shape our destiny through how we live.

In this chapter I will explain how joyspan affects your lifespan by delving into the difference between lifespan and life expectancy, the detrimental impact of the antiaging culture, what you do and do not have control over, and research on how psychological well-being affects lifespan.

LIFESPAN VS. LIFE EXPECTANCY

When people talk about aging, they tend to use the terms "lifespan" and "life expectancy" interchangeably, but they are not the same thing. Here is a breakdown of what each term means, how they differ, and why these differences are important for understanding your mortality.

Lifespan is the total amount of time an individual or a species can live, measured from birth to death. This concept can be applied to individuals, populations, or species, and reflects the *potential* maximum duration of life. Maximum lifespan is the longest recorded age reached by any individual of a species. In humans, the oldest verified person as of this writing was Jeanne Calment, a French woman who lived 122 years and 164 days.[3] Maximum lifespan means the biological limits of human longevity, shaped by factors like genetics, cellular aging, and environmental constraints. Lifespan is focused on the total number of years lived, and in its purest form, it is about the limits of human biology and survival.

Studies have put the human lifespan limit somewhere between 125 and 150 years. Researchers in Singapore, Russia, and the United States used a computer model to estimate that the limit of human lifespan is about 150 years. These researchers took blood samples from more than seventy thousand participants up to age eighty-five and looked at short-term changes in their blood cell counts. The number of white blood cells a person has can indicate the level of inflammation in their body, while the volume of red blood cells can indicate a person's risk of heart disease or stroke, as well as cognitive impairment, such as memory loss. These calculations predicted that for everyone—regardless of their health or genetics—resilience failed completely at 150, giving a theoretical limit to the human lifespan.[4] But before you start planning for your 150-year-long life, keep in mind that it is a theoretical model.

Life expectancy is a statistical measure of how long a person or population is expected to live, based on historical data and current conditions. It is an average prediction rather than an individual outcome and reflects trends in mortality at specific ages or over time. Life expectancy is calculated using mortality rates across age groups to predict how long, on average, a person is expected to live. The formula accounts for factors like infant mortality, accidents, and chronic diseases that affect survival rates at different life stages. Life expectancy varies by geographic region, sex, and socioeconomic status. Globally, the human life expectancy is seventy-three. There is considerable variability in average life expectancy by country, though, with Japan at 85 years, New Zealand at 84 years, Canada at 83 years, the United Kingdom at 81 years, the United States at 79 years, Mexico at 76 years, Russia at 73 years, and Chad at 54 years.[5]

Life expectancy changes with age because with each age you attain, you've avoided causes of death. Dr. Marie Bernard, former deputy director of the National Institute on Aging at the National Institutes of Health, explained, "If you make it to age 65, the likelihood that you'll make it to 85 is very high. And if you make it to 85, the likelihood that you'll make it to 92 is very high."[6]

Across the world, women live an average of five years longer than men. Globally, the average life expectancy is seventy-four years for women versus sixty-eight years for men. The gender gap in life expectancy begins at birth: Newborn boys have higher death rates than newborn girls, as they're more vulnerable to diseases and genetic disorders. The gap continues in youth, when boys have a higher death rate than girls, typically due to violence and accidents. As we grow older, men have higher death rates than women from chronic health conditions, which are partly due to higher rates of smoking, alcohol, and drug use. In the past, gender differences in infant mortality were the leading cause of the disparity in life expectancy. But now, differences at older ages are a larger contributor to the gap in life expectancy.[7] The small, everyday choices we make in our lives impact our life expectancies and they matter at every age and stage.

Inequality in life expectancy exists not only by gender but also by socioeconomic status and racial disparities. People of color have consistently had a lower life expectancy, and the COVID-19 pandemic exacerbated this fact. Reducing these disparities is literally a matter of life and death. To improve life expectancy across communities, we need to reduce inequalities in health insurance, increase access

KEY DIFFERENCES BETWEEN LIFESPAN AND LIFE EXPECTANCY

	Lifespan	*Life Expectancy*
Definition	Total number of years a person lives	Predicted average number of years a person will live
Measurement	Individual or biological limit of survival	Statistical average for a population or cohort
Scope	Focuses on maximum potential (how long life can last)	Focuses on average outcomes (how long people are likely to live)
Example	Jeanne Calment lived to 122 years.	In 2024, life expectancy at birth: 64.1 in Africa 72.3 in Russia 73.5 in Mexico 79.1 in the United States 81.7 in the United Kingdom 82.8 in New Zealand 85 in Japan*

* World Bank (2024). *Life expectancy at birth, total (years)* [Data file]. Retrieved from https://data.worldbank.org/indicator/SP.DYN.LE00.IN.

(continued)

	Lifespan	*Life Expectancy*
Determinants	Biological and lifestyle factors	Biological and lifestyle factors *and* health care, public health, socioeconomic factors
Predictive Value	Not predictive—looks at achieved lifespans	Predictive—estimates future survival rates
Unit of Analysis	Individual or species	Population or cohort
Implication for Policy	Highlights the biological limit of longevity	Informs public health strategies to increase survival

to care, and eliminate discrimination and bias. Beyond the healthcare system, this includes tackling economic stability, neighborhood and physical environment, education, food security, and community safety. A society is judged in part by how it treats older adults and the place it gives them in community life. Until everyone can maximize the length of their life, we have not succeeded.

Lifespan and life expectancy are both about how many years you will live: quantity. These are important numbers because to live a *good* long life, you need to, well, live. But a long lifespan is not the end of the story. With all the focus upon quantity of life, the *quality* of life, or joyspan, has been overshadowed—especially when it comes to the multibillion-dollar antiaging industry.

OUR ANTIAGING CULTURE

The antiaging noise is deafening. We are bombarded with the message that growing old is unacceptable, something we must try to stop. We are urged to swallow the latest supplements, slough off dead skin cells, smear on facial serums, do cold plunges, take warm saunas, and exercise at 0 dark hundred. Antiaging sells by generating fear and insecurity, and the brainwashing starts early. We're fed a steady diet of "Older is ugly and scary" messaging from toddlerhood. One of my earliest memories was how scared I was of the old woman in the story "Snow White and the Seven Dwarfs." She was an evil witch who created a poisonous apple to give to the little girl. In the picture book I studied the warts on her nose, her sharp nails, and her scowling expression. At three years old, message received: Old is bad. Don't get old.

We live in a society that worships youth, fresh faces, lithe bodies, the new, the cool, the hip. Greeting cards are full of put-downs about being older, older characters on TV are depicted as bumbling idiots, and everywhere you turn the message hammered into us is that young is good and old is bad.

Prejudice on the grounds of a person's age—*ageism*—is the last acceptable form of discrimination. Only it isn't acceptable.

The antiaging industry is based on convincing us that we are not okay as we are. Our skin is not tight enough; our teeth are too yellow; we are too flabby, not radiant enough, not young enough. Enough for what? The goal is to elicit enough fear to cause you to act and try to buy youth. Global spending on antiaging products and treatments is significant and growing. In 2024, the market was estimated to reach approximately $68 billion, driven by increasing awareness and consumer demand for solutions addressing wrinkles, skin rejuvenation, and hair restoration. Projections indicate the market will expand further, potentially reaching $141 billion by 2034.[8] We spend billions every year to try to be worthy of love and respect. The reality is that we are already worthy of love and respect.

Do you remember how old you were when you first experienced ageism? I do!

During COVID, our three grown kids had returned home. Amid

Zoom meetings and wiping down groceries, our twenty-one-year-old daughter, Claire, offered to teach us a dance. Wearing tie-dyed pants and a colorful T-shirt, I danced until sweat poured down my face. She then posted our dance video on social media. All the comments were along these lines:

"OMG, how cute your mom is—hilarious." Cute? Hilarious? The comment wasn't about the dancing, it was about my age—I was in my early fifties. I was seen as a silly older person doing a dance. As I was reading these comments, I accidentally flipped the phone camera around and got an extreme close-up of my face and neck. Oh, the chins!

My internalized ageism was telling me how unacceptable and unattractive it was that my skin bunched up under my chin. I decided to record a video about ageism and posted it on social media. Despite having only a handful of followers, half a million people watched it and thousands of comments poured in.

"I can't stand that I'm losing my looks."

"I'm terrified to think what lies ahead."

"Getting old sucks."

Fear was the common denominator. The most damaging aspect of living in an ageist society is how we turn the ageist beliefs inward. Ageism becomes internalized ageism. We all live with internalized ageism. Once you start to become aware of it, you hear it everywhere. Just yesterday, a friend said, "I hate getting old, watching it all slide, my body, my looks, my ability to do it all." She had internalized the belief that young is good and old is bad. She believes that since she is no longer young, she is no longer...good. We accept the assertion that old is weak, unattractive, less than. These beliefs are not limited to our external selves but extend to the core of who we are—our competence, our value, our relevance. On TV, in movies, or in greeting cards, older people are depicted as tottering, blathering, clueless, grumpy, selfish, and embarrassing. Those messages and images take root within us and provide a negative guide as we grow older. Now *we* are the tottering, blathering, clueless, grumpy, selfish, and embarrassing side characters. This mindset leads us to limit our aspirations, goals, and opportunities. We refrain from pursuing new interests and advancements because we believe that we are no longer capable or relevant.

Recognizing how pervasive and harmful ageism is will help you break free of the self-fulfilling prophecy of internalized ageism. It's a bit like seeing behind the curtain in *The Wizard of Oz*. Pull back the antiaging veil, and you will see companies who trade on fear. With heightened awareness, you will start to notice when people around you fall for it. You will hear comments such as "I am showing my age," or "I am having a senior moment," in a different way. Advertisements of young women obsessing about their skin will seem like a waste of precious time. Rather than compliment someone for looking "young," you will see that "young" needn't be the goal. You'll skip the antiaging birthday cards. You will reclaim your age, reclaim your life.

But be forewarned, you will face a powerful current of people swimming in the other direction. People spending their lives trying not to age, trying not to die. Why not try to live instead?

———— JOY PRACTICE: ————
Test Your Own Ageist Beliefs

For each question, choose the option that best reflects your belief.

You are coming upon a milestone birthday; how are you feeling?

    a. Argh!! I feel sick about the thought of being this old.
    b. I don't love it, but it's not the end of the world.
    c. I'm getting ready to celebrate.

If you hear a friend describe an older person as cute, what do you think?

    a. I wouldn't think anything of it; old people are so cute.
    b. I can see it might sound a bit patronizing, but it's not meant with any harm.
    c. It is patronizing and I don't say that.

How do you feel about antiaging marketing?

    a. Great! To look good, we need products to cover up the signs of aging.
    b. That marketing isn't ideal, but people do want to look young.
    c. People don't need to fight aging; it's a natural process and looking good does not need to mean looking young.

Do you use any of these phrases?: You can't teach an old dog new tricks; I'm too old for this, I'm having a senior moment; You look good . . . for your age.

    a. I sure do!
    b. I seldom do.
    c. I never do.

RESULTS

MOSTLY "a." ANSWERS:

Uh-oh, you hold negative views toward aging that you may want to examine and adjust. Endorsing a negative view of aging has been shown to result in a reduction of seven to ten years of life.

MOSTLY "b." ANSWERS:

You may have some biases to examine in order to free yourself from ageism.

MOSTLY "C." ANSWERS:

You value older adults and see aging positively. Great! This will impact both the length and the quality of your life.

HOW JOYSPAN IMPROVES LIFESPAN

An innovative and seminal study in gerontology sought to show how joyspan improves lifespan by tracking the physical, cognitive, and emotional health of 180 nuns over their lifetimes. Lead researcher David Snowdon and his team analyzed autobiographical essays the nuns wrote in their early twenties. Results showed that the nuns who conveyed gratitude, enthusiasm, and joy lived on average seven to ten years longer than those who expressed neutral or negative emotions. The findings demonstrated that one's emotional outlook in youth has long-term effects, possibly building psychological resilience against chronic stressors. Interestingly, even when lifestyle factors such as smoking and alcohol consumption were controlled, the positive effect of emotional well-being remained a strong predictor of longevity. The nun study highlights that joyspan—the cultivation of continued growth, social connection, generosity, and adaptability—acts as a buffer against cognitive decline and supports health well into old age.[9]

These findings were replicated by a larger and longer longitudinal study, the Harvard Study of Adult Development. Researchers tracked the lives of two groups—Harvard sophomores and inner-city Boston men—over eighty years, analyzing the impacts of various life factors on health and happiness. Social connection played a more significant role in predicting lifespan than socioeconomic status, wealth, or professional success. Those with strong social bonds and joyful relationships also exhibited lower levels of stress hormones, such as cortisol, which are known to accelerate aging and damage cardiovascular health. Conversely, loneliness and emotional distress were found to increase the risk of early mortality.[10]

Building upon these landmark studies, a large meta-analysis of studies found that people who regularly experience positive emotions tend to engage in healthier behaviors, including exercise, balanced diets, and better sleep routines. These individuals are also more likely to maintain strong social relationships. Positive emotions reduce the production of stress-related hormones, improve immune system functioning, and enhance cardiovascular performance. By fostering emotional resilience, happiness helps individuals cope with adversity more effectively, minimizing the health risks associated with chronic stress.[11] The cumulative effect of frequent positive affects creates a joyspan, which not only improves day-to-day life but also contributes to a longer lifespan.

Here are the main mechanisms through which joyspan can influence lifespan.

Stronger Social Connections

Relationships are a key component of joy. People with strong social ties—whether through friendships, family, or community—experience more joy and meaning in life. Loneliness and social isolation are significant predictors of early mortality, with research showing they are as harmful to health as smoking fifteen cigarettes a day.[12] Social connections improve emotional well-being and act as a buffer against stress, encouraging people to live longer, healthier lives.

Resilience and Coping

As people age, they encounter challenges such as health problems, the loss of loved ones, and reduced physical abilities. Joyful individuals exhibit greater emotional resilience, helping them recover from setbacks more easily. Resilience protects mental health, reducing the risk of depression and anxiety, which are linked to poorer health outcomes and shorter lifespans. Resilient people stay engaged with life even in difficult times, leading to greater life satisfaction and longevity.

Slower Cognitive Decline

Joyful living contributes to better cognitive health by promoting mental engagement, curiosity, and social interaction. Positive emotions help protect the brain from cognitive decline, reducing the risk of Alzheimer's and other forms of dementia. Maintaining purpose and meaning—important aspects of joyspan—has been shown to improve cognitive longevity, keeping the mind sharp well into old age.

HOW TO CULTIVATE JOY TO IMPROVE YOUR LIFESPAN

Gratitude practice: Regularly reflecting on things you are thankful for enhances emotional well-being.
Exercise and play: Physical activity releases endorphins, improving mood and increasing joy.
Social connections: Nurture friendships and family relationships to build emotional resilience.
Mindfulness and meditation: These practices reduce stress and increase present-moment joy.
Meaningful work and hobbies: Engage in activities that bring purpose and fulfillment.
Acts of kindness: Helping others generates a lasting sense of joy and connection.
Laughter: Spend time with people or engage in activities that make you laugh—laughter has measurable health benefits.

THE DOWNSIDE OF A LONG LIFE WITHOUT JOYSPAN

Even if we can't live forever, advances in medicine, public health, and lifestyle choices have extended our lifespans. For far too many, a longer life just means more suffering. Jill C. lived to be ninety-four years old and is a reminder that longevity alone does not guarantee a meaningful or satisfying life.

Jill and George married in their twenties and raised their three children together. Jill often felt more like a manager than a mother, ensuring that everyone was fed, clothed, and on time. Jill shared that her marriage lacked emotional intimacy but that she didn't put in the time to foster really close friendships with other women. When their children moved away, she didn't find new interests or activities to fill the void. Instead, she spent her days cleaning, cooking, and watching television alone in the evenings.

"As I grew older, I wondered, what else is there?" she told me in her late eighties.

Jill's emotional isolation worsened as the years went by. She avoided conversations about feelings, even with her grown children, who found her distant and difficult. When friends or family expressed any feelings, Jill felt like a disconnected spectator. She neglected her emotional well-being, and her joyspan was far shorter than both her healthspan and her lifespan.

By the time she reached her seventies, she no longer heard from two of her children. Her youngest son visited out of obligation, but they were not close either. After her husband's death, her days were monotonous, marked only by visits to the grocery store and medical appointments. She resisted joining community activities because that "seemed desperate." When I asked what she meant by that she explained that she saw membership groups as forced friends for people who didn't have friends, a take that is as inaccurate as it is self-limiting.

Her long life gave her ample time to reflect, but instead of joy or gratitude, Jill was filled with regret. She regretted not pursuing her passion for painting, a joy she abandoned in her thirties. She regretted not expressing love more freely to her children and not building meaningful friendships. Even in the face of these regrets, Jill did not opt for change or growth. She told herself, "It's too late now."

Though she lived into her nineties, Jill's life was not enriched by her extra years. Her physical health remained relatively good, but her emotional well-being was in constant decline. She avoided joy as if it were a luxury she couldn't afford, even though joy was the one thing that might have made her long life meaningful.

THE IMPACT OF A LONG LIFE WITHOUT JOY

Loneliness and Isolation

The World Health Organization warns that loneliness and social isolation are among the leading causes of poor mental health in older populations. Older individuals who lack meaningful relationships are at a higher risk of depression and cognitive impairment, with some studies showing that loneliness increases mortality risk by 26 percent.[13] Without interventions to foster social engagement, longer lifespans may lead to more years of emotional suffering.

Mental Health Decline

A long life lived without joy has significant mental health repercussions. Depression is prevalent among older adults, and many do not receive adequate mental health care due to stigma, limited access, or underdiagnosis. The psychological impact of feeling "left behind" in a rapidly evolving world, along with diminished social roles and ageism, can result in decreased self-worth and despair. As individuals grow older without meaningful engagement, their risk for mental health disorders such as anxiety and suicidal ideation increases.

Economic Strain

Beyond health-care expenses, the economic cost of unfulfilled aging includes the loss of contributions from older adults who could otherwise engage in productive or voluntary activities. Encouraging lifelong learning, community involvement, and intergenerational interaction can help mitigate these losses. However, without addressing the emotional needs of older adults, their potential contributions remain untapped, limiting society's ability to benefit from their experience and wisdom.

The greatest downside of a long life without joyspan is suffering. For Jill, and so many others like her, small changes in factors known to increase psychological well-being could have resulted in significantly more joy. Things that you can do today will impact your well-being in longevity. In charting your second half of life, you won't have control over everything, but you'll have more than you think.

WHAT YOU DO AND DO NOT HAVE CONTROL OVER WHEN IT COMES TO LIFESPAN

Human lifespan is determined by a complex interplay between genetic, environmental, and lifestyle factors. While certain aspects are within our control, others are governed by biology and chance.

People love to blame genes, but the truth is that genes are not the most important part of the equation for most of us. Genes are responsible for around 25 percent of the variation in lifespan and the remaining 75 percent is the result of our beliefs, attitudes, choices, and behaviors.[14] The key to life expectancy and healthy aging is to engage fully in life—mentally, physically, socially, and emotionally.

What Is Not Under Your Control

Genetic Factors

Genetics plays a relatively small role in predicting how long you'll live, but it does play a part. Genes involved in repairing DNA, regulating metabolism, and managing oxidative stress influence longevity and how well the body ages. For example, variants in the FOXO3 gene have been associated with exceptional longevity by improving cellular repair mechanisms and stress responses.[15]

Biological Aging

Aging is an unavoidable biological process, driven by cellular aging, declining stem cell function, and cumulative molecular damage.

Accidents and Random Events

Unpredictable occurrences, including accidents, natural disasters, and sudden medical events, such as strokes or cardiac arrest, also affect lifespan. These events fall outside personal control and can occur despite the best health practices. In fact, studies show that external risks, particularly in the form of sudden trauma, account for a small but significant portion of premature deaths worldwide.

Environmental Exposures

Although you can make conscious efforts to reduce exposure to harmful pollutants, environmental risks cannot be completely avoided. Air quality, water contamination, and exposure to infectious agents all have measurable impacts on health and lifespan. For example, long-term exposure to air pollution increases the risk of respiratory diseases and reduces life expectancy by several years.[16] The COVID-19 pandemic demonstrated how pathogens, even in highly developed societies, can drastically reduce life expectancy on a global scale.

What Is Under Your Control

Your Social Connections

Loneliness is a risk factor for early mortality. Loneliness increases stress-related hormones like cortisol. The Harvard Study of Adult Development revealed that quality relationships is one of the most important predictors of longevity and well-being. People with strong social connections experience lower levels of stress hormones, reduced inflammation, and better cardiovascular health. Social activities and group involvement have also been linked to lower risks of depression and dementia in older adults.[17]

YOUR SOCIAL CONNECTIONS ACTION ITEMS

- Be proactive in cultivating and maintaining social connections.
- Engage in group activities such as volunteering, clubs, or classes.
- Pursue lifelong learning to challenge your brain and connect with other people who are interested in ongoing growth.

Your Attitude

Your attitude significantly impacts your lifespan. Yale researcher Dr. Becca Levy found that individuals with positive self-perceptions of aging live years longer than those with negative perceptions.[18] How you view your life's purpose also impacts your lifespan. In Japan, "*ikigai*," or a sense of purpose in life, has been linked to lower mortality rates in Japanese populations. Purposeful living not only motivates individuals to engage in healthier behaviors but also buffers against stress and reduces the risk of depression and anxiety. Optimism, another key factor, has been associated with improved immune function and lower mortality from heart disease and stroke.[19]

> **YOUR ATTITUDE ACTION ITEMS**
>
> - Cultivate a sense of purpose by setting meaningful goals.
> - Practice gratitude and mindfulness to foster a positive mindset.
> - Engage in community involvement, hobbies, or work that provides fulfillment.

Your Smoking and Alcohol Consumption

Avoiding tobacco and limiting alcohol consumption are powerful steps you can take to increase your lifespan. Smoking remains a leading cause of preventable death, responsible for eight million deaths annually, according to the World Health Organization. The good news is that quitting smoking yields immediate and long-term benefits. Within twenty-four hours, blood pressure normalizes, and within a few weeks, lung function begins to improve. Even individuals who quit smoking later in life experience significant health improvements, including a 40 percent reduction in cardiovascular mortality within five years of quitting.[20]

Excessive alcohol consumption is linked to increased risks of liver disease, cancer, and cognitive decline. The safest strategy for longevity is to limit or avoid alcohol altogether, as even moderate drinking can increase the risk of certain cancers.

> ### YOUR SUBSTANCE USE ACTION ITEMS
>
> - Quit smoking: Use evidence-based strategies such as nicotine replacement therapy, behavioral counseling, or medications like bupropion, a drug prescribed to help people quit smoking.
> - Alcohol moderation: Limit alcohol intake to within recommended guidelines or explore nonalcoholic alternatives.
> - Avoid secondhand smoke: Prolonged exposure increases the risk of heart disease by 25 to 30 percent even in nonsmokers.*
>
> ---
> *U.S. Department of Health and Human Services (2006). *The health consequences of involuntary exposure to tobacco smoke: A report of the Surgeon General.* Centers for Disease Control and Prevention.

The key to optimizing lifespan lies in focusing on modifiable factors. Although genetics and aging processes are beyond individual control, lifestyle choices like diet, exercise, and stress management can add both years to life and life to years. Additionally, fostering strong social bonds and participating in preventive health care further boost longevity. Dr. Pinchas Cohen, dean of the Leonard Davis School of Gerontology at the University of Southern California, says that living longer in the future is certainly possible; over the course of the twentieth century, human life expectancy rose from around age fifty to more than eighty years. But he continues, "Death is not optional; it's written into our genes. There's absolutely no evidence that [living forever] is possible, and there's absolutely no technology right now that even suggests that we're heading there."[21]

Scientific advancements may, in the future, extend our control over biological aging, but for now, practical habits remain the best tools we have.

TRYING TO BEAT AGING

Bryan Johnson is a forty-seven-year-old tech entrepreneur who spends more than $2 million a year on his antiaging protocol. He eats dinner at 11:30 a.m., goes to bed at 8:30 p.m., takes no vacations in the sun, eats meticulously crafted diets, works out for hours per day, and receives plasma infusions, undergoes high-tech medical tests, and takes in excess of one hundred supplements every day.

According to Johnson, "Most people assume death is inevitable. Not anymore." While Johnson's commitment and resources are extreme, he is not alone in his zealous pursuit of youth. In 2024, he hosted the Don't Die Summit, which attracted over ten thousand attendees, in ten cities, at $170–$599 per ticket. Featured discussions and activities included cryotherapy, intravenous nutrient drips, genetic testing, sleep optimization, and microdosing psychedelics.

Hype aside, is it possible to reject aging and avoid death? Even if we could live forever, would we want to?

THE KEY TO LONGER LIFE EXPECTANCY

Why did identical twins Josephine and Janice experience such different lifespans despite their identical genetics? Their joyspans impacted their lifespans, and vice versa. Born minutes apart, their early years were filled with the same laughter and mischief. As they grew, subtle differences began to emerge in their emotional resilience, attitudes, and approaches to life that would eventually determine the very shape of their lives.

In elementary school, Josephine was optimistic and curious. She loved school, not because it came easily, but because she liked learning and had fun with the other kids. When faced with difficult subjects, Josephine would ask questions and reach out to teachers for help. Janice approached challenges with fear and frustration. She withdrew from academic difficulties and saw failures as personal shortcomings. While Josephine joined clubs and made friends easily, Janice felt left out.

These patterns grew as the girls got older. Josephine leaned into connection, growth, and adaptability (see figure 5), while Janice grew more rigid and critical.

After high school, Josephine pursued nursing and thrived in the busy hospital environment, where every day was different. She embraced change, and when things didn't go her way, she adjusted. Her openness and generosity extended to her colleagues, who admired her disposition even during stressful shifts.

Janice held several office jobs but felt unfulfilled. She stayed on in positions she didn't enjoy. At work, she kept to herself. While Josephine found purpose in her career, Janice saw work as a necessary evil. Over time, her attitude wore her down, contributing to chronic stress and dissatisfaction.

Josephine's warmth translated into deep friendships. She maintained close connections with friends from childhood, nursing school, and even neighbors from different stages of life. These friendships provided a rich tapestry of support, laughter, and meaning. She would host small gatherings and made herself available when a friend was in need.

Janice struggled to form lasting friendships. Though she envied

Josephine's social circle, she often felt others were judging her. Her insecurity caused her to pull away. When friends reached out, she declined invitations and, over time, her social world shrank.

In their later years, the sisters' differences became even more apparent. Josephine remained active well into her eighties and nineties. Even as her body slowed, she found joy in small things—a good book, a sunset, or a cup of tea with a friend. When her eyesight began to deteriorate, she switched to audiobooks. When arthritis made it difficult to garden, she planted herbs in small indoor pots. She approached aging as an opportunity to explore new ways of living fully.

Janice's pessimism and rigidity increased as she grew older. When arthritis made it difficult to move, she stopped exercising altogether. She developed diabetes in her sixties and struggled with heart disease in her seventies. Janice died at age seventy-eight, after years of battling dementia and chronic illnesses. At Janice's memorial service, Josephine was one of four people in attendance.

FIGURE 5. Joyspan Matrix in Action: Josephine, Age 97

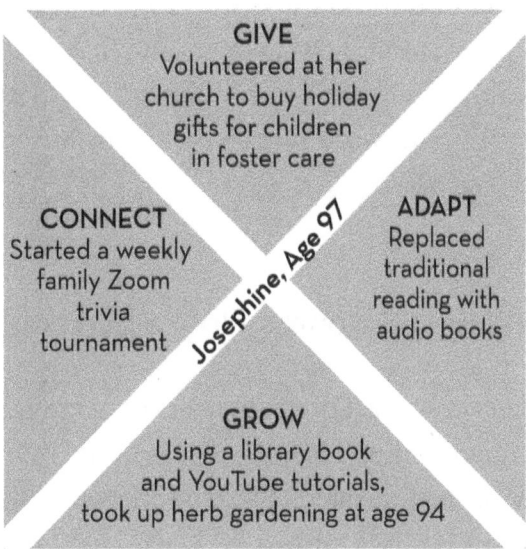

Josephine lived independently until the end, passing in her sleep at ninety-seven. Her friends and family gathered to celebrate her life, sharing stories of her kindness, humor, and generosity. "She made the world brighter," one of her grandsons said during the eulogy. Her home was filled with small reminders of a life well-lived—her paintings, books she had loved, and photographs of friends and family.

Josephine enjoyed a joyspan as long as her ninety-seven-year lifespan.

——— JOY PRACTICE: ———
Self-Reflection Exercise

For this exercise, grab your journal. Draw a line down the middle of a page, and in the left column, create a list of reasons you would like to live as long as possible if you could. On the right column, list the reasons you *don't* necessarily want to live much longer. Be as honest and specific as you can. Study your lists and ask yourself what assumptions you are making on both sides. Is this a different list than you would have created at age twenty? Will your list still look the same at age ninety?

This chapter examined how joyspan increases years of life. In the next chapter, we examine how joyspan also increases the years of life in good health. Contentment, fulfillment, and purpose not only enrich life but also add years to it—a win-win for both emotional well-being and longevity.

JOYSPANNER: Baroness Floella Benjamin

Baroness Benjamin is a Trinidadian-British actress, singer, presenter, author and politician who was born 1949. In the 1970s and 80s, she presented children's television, including *Play School*, but has now turned her attention to politics.

In 2020 she was named in the Powerlist's the Top 100 most influential people in the UK of African/African-Caribbean descent.

- **GROW:** In the last two decades, Floella has campaigned on issues related to children's welfare. In 2010 she became the first actress to become a Peer in the UK's House of Lords.
- **CONNECT:** Connection and helping others is of paramount importance to Baroness Benjamin. Speaking to RedOnline, she said: 'I'm a firm believer that when you give, give, give, you haven't got time to feel mentally depressed or strained.'
- **ADAPT:** Floella has often talked about needing to keep fit as her body gets older. She does sit ups and leg exercises daily, as well as regular stretching.
- **GIVE:** Floella has been tireless campaigner for children's issues, working with a number of charities including Barnardo's and the NSPCC. She has also spoken out against racism and championed diversity, trying to inspire people to do better.

Floella's dedication to her purpose empowering children is both inspiring and impressive, as is her attitude to aging. By using her platform as a children's TV presenter, she has managed to bring about real change.

CHAPTER 3

How Your Joyspan Affects Your Healthspan

Betty was an only child. Throughout her life she longed for a sibling and envied the closeness of sisters. She imagined sharing secrets and clothes and having someone to lean on throughout life. In college, she found what she had been searching for in Lynn. The two became inseparable and Lynn became the sister my mother had always wanted.

Betty and Lynn each married, and they both had three children, whom they raised side by side. The friends shared bake sales, college send-offs, children's weddings, and parents' funerals. They were similar in most ways. One small difference between them became deeply significant over time. Betty was mindful of daily health decisions—nothing extreme, just thoughtful. Lynn, on the other hand, opted for whatever was easiest. She skipped workouts, ate processed food, favored Cokes to water, and didn't bother with regular doctor check-ups or dental cleanings.

Betty is not a health fanatic. She loves a slice of pie or the occasional dry martini. But she is vigilant about certain habits. She stretches each morning, cooks healthy meals, takes daily walks, slathers on sunscreen, and keeps up with dental and medical appointments.

Lynn felt like life was too short to fuss over such things. If she wanted dessert, she'd eat the whole slice, and probably a second. Sunscreen, water intake, exercise, and doctor appointments weren't a priority. She'd chide Betty, saying, "Aw c'mon, live a little. You really think one more little whatever (cola, slice of cake, cigarette) matters?" For many years, the differences in their habits didn't seem to be significant. They were both healthy and happy, and to me "Aunt Lynn" seemed cooler as a result of her relaxed approach.

By the time Betty and Lynn reached their sixties, small differences began to emerge, almost imperceptibly at first. Betty's energy remained steady—she still walked most mornings, stayed active in her garden, and looked forward to tennis with her friends. She wasn't without her share of aches and pains, but she managed them and stuck to her routines.

Lynn, on the other hand, started to slow down in her sixties. A nagging stiffness in her joints turned into chronic pain. Her energy waned, until getting up off the couch or going to the grocery store felt exhausting. "I just need to rest more," she'd say when Betty invited her out. Lynn's body was catching up with her choices.

For both Betty and Lynn, the little things accumulated over time—to the benefit of Betty and the detriment of Lynn. When they reached their late seventies, Lynn could no longer walk or transfer from her chair to her bed or to the restroom, and she required full-time care. Lynn passed away shortly after her eightieth birthday. Although her lifespan was eighty years, her healthspan was seventy years. On the other hand, Betty is now ninety-six and still going strong.

But what about their joyspans? Lynn's joyspan was shorter than Betty's. Lynn's joyspan was around seventy-two years as compared to ninety-six years and counting for Betty. Lynn's reduced healthspan impacted her joyspan in the final years of her life, as she lived with a great deal of pain and shortness of breath.

WHAT IS HEALTHSPAN?

Healthspan is the amount of life spent in good health. Lifespan is the *quantity* of years and healthspan is the *quality of those years*. Healthspan is often thought of as being about the physical, but physical health is only one-third of the health equation. Your healthspan encompasses your physical health, your cognitive health, and your emotional health. All three are crucially important, intertwined, and dependent upon one another. To extend healthspan, you need to give your cognitive and emotional health the same attention that you give to your physical health.

This section explores all three aspects of healthspan by reviewing what's normal and how to be proactive when it comes to your physical, cognitive, and emotional health in longevity.

PHYSICAL CHANGES: WHAT'S NORMAL AS YOU GROW OLDER?

Your muscles. You lose about 10 to 15 percent of your muscle mass and strength over your lifetime. Muscle loss happens because of a reduction in muscle-building hormones and changes to your muscle fibers. Severe muscle loss, sarcopenia, is *not* a natural part of aging. It's often the result of a lack of physical activity or another health problem. The condition affects as many as 13 percent of people ages sixty to seventy. That number goes up to 50 percent after age eighty.[1] The good news is that you can avoid or delay a lot of age-related muscle loss. The key is regular resistance, or strength, training. If you maintain your strength, you're more likely to live independently, fall less, and recover from serious injuries faster.

Your bones. At every age, our bones break down and rebuild daily.

When you reach middle age, the breakdown happens faster than bones can rebuild and they can become more fragile. Bone weakness is more common in everyone starting at age fifty, but your odds of low bone mass are higher if you're female because of drops in estrogen. Female bones are also smaller and less dense than male bones. Older people are more likely to develop osteopenia, or low bone mass, which can be an early warning sign of osteoporosis, a condition where your bones are very weak and can break easily. Talk to your doctor about bone loss. You might not have any symptoms until you get hurt. In general, you should get your bone density checked starting at age sixty-five if you're a woman and seventy if you're a man.

Your senses. It is normal for the lens in your eyes to harden, which makes it difficult to focus on objects close-up, such as menus. It is also normal to experience some hearing loss, especially with high-frequency sounds. Both visual and hearing impairment can impact not only the quality of life but also your cognition. So it is important to have routine eye exams and hearing tests for early intervention to correct vision with glasses or contacts and hearing with hearing aids.

Your skin. Skin becomes thinner and less elastic over time. We make less collagen and elastin and lose fat in certain areas. Bruises and scratches may take longer to heal. You also sweat less as you age. You might not be able to cool yourself off quickly if you get hot. Skin cancer is the most common type of cancer, so check yourself for new or unusual moles or freckles or other growths and have your doctor check you as well.

Your heart. It is normal for the shape and strength of your heart and blood vessels to change over time. Blood vessels get thicker and stiffer with age. That makes it harder to push blood through your body. Your blood pressure might go up or not stabilize as quickly. The aging process doesn't cause heart and blood vessel problems for everyone, however. High blood pressure is the most common heart condition for people seventy-five and older. And heart disease is the leading cause of death for both men and women. Symptoms of heart disease include shortness of breath, chest pains, or feeling like your heart skips a beat. Tell your doctor if you experience these symptoms.

Your digestive system. Your metabolism slows as you age. It is also common for muscles in your lower throat to weaken so the flap that keeps food in your stomach might pop open more often, resulting in heartburn. Compared to when you were younger, your blood sugar might spike more after a meal. That's not a big deal usually, but unmanaged high blood sugar can lead to diabetes. Food might move through your intestines a little slower, which leads to constipation. For these common changes, it is critical to stay hydrated, eat plenty of fiber, and get enough physical activity.

PHYSICAL HEALTH: WHAT YOU CAN DO

- **Regular exercise:** Aim to move your body every day. Get a least thirty to sixty minutes of moderate to vigorous aerobic exercise five days a week (e.g., walking, swimming, cycling, dancing). Work on your strength two or more days per week (e.g., weights, resistance bands, push-ups, squats), and work on your balance and flexibility two to three times per week (e.g., yoga, balance exercises).[2] If you want to feel well, you need to make all three types of exercise a habit. If you don't stretch, your body will tighten up, making it hard to walk. If you don't work on muscle strength, you'll lose muscle and have a hard time getting out of a chair. If you don't get aerobic exercise (walk, bike, swim, dance, etc.), your heart will grow weaker, and you'll always be tired.
- **Nutrition:** Chose nutrient-rich meals and snacks. Fruits, vegetables, whole grains, healthy fats, and quality proteins can lower the risk of chronic diseases. Adequate protein intake is crucial for muscle maintenance. If you are fifty or older, aim for an intake of 1.0–1.5 grams of protein per kilogram of body weight

to help maintain muscle mass and prevent age-related muscle loss.[3] Getting a good mix of protein sources—lean meats, fish, eggs, dairy, beans, and plant-based sources—can help make sure you get both protein and other essential nutrients.
- **Sleep:** Sleep experts advise us to get seven to eight hours of sleep each night to support our physical recovery, cognition, and mental health. The research is powerful, but the reality is that many of us struggle with sleep as we grow older. Getting sunlight in the morning has been shown to help, as does limiting caffeine, as well as creating a bedtime ritual (in a dark, quiet, cool room).
- **Preventive health care:** Scheduling regular checkups with health-care and dental professionals goes a long way in identifying health risks. For many conditions, early intervention makes all the difference.

COGNITIVE CHANGES: WHAT'S NORMAL AS YOU GROW OLDER?

Cognitive health is your ability to think, learn, and remember effectively. Research shows that certain cognitive abilities, particularly those related to accumulated knowledge and experience, often remain stable or even improve with age. Vocabulary, for example, tends to increase with age, as older adults continue to acquire and use new words over time. This is supported by longitudinal studies that demonstrate older adults often perform better on vocabulary tests compared to younger adults.[4] Creativity and reasoning, particularly in areas requiring insight and life experience, can also strengthen with age. With age we get better at what researchers call "wise reasoning," which involves recognizing others' perspectives, acknowledging the variability of life, and dealing with social conflicts in ways that are beneficial to long-term social harmony.[5]

Other parts of the brain, such as your processing speed and recall, tend to decline with age. It is normal for our brains to lose mass as we grow older. It's also normal for our brains to receive less blood flow, and the connections between nerve cells slows. These age-related changes may have some unwanted side effects. For example, your attention span might get a little shorter and some things might be harder to recall. You may find yourself searching for words and experiencing that "on-the-tip-of-the-tongue" feeling. Memory slips can feel scary but don't necessarily mean you will experience cognitive impairment.

Also known as dementia, cognitive impairment is *not* a normal part of aging. "Dementia" is an umbrella term used to describe a collection of symptoms that a person may experience from a variety of diseases including Alzheimer's disease, vascular dementia, Lewy body dementia, frontotemporal dementia, and Huntington's disease. Dementia is often referred to as "senility" or "senile dementia," which reflects the incorrect belief that serious memory decline is a normal part of aging. Though dementia is not a normal part of aging, it's more common as people get older. Globally, dementia affects around 5 to 7 percent of people age sixty and older, with rates climbing to nearly 40 percent among those over age ninety.[6] Factors proved to increase the risk of developing dementia are: age, high blood pressure (hypertension), high blood sugar (diabetes), being overweight, smoking, drinking too much alcohol, being physically inactive, being socially isolated, and depression.[7]

COGNITIVE HEALTH: WHAT YOU CAN DO

Here's what you can do to improve your cognitive health and lower your risk for cognitive impairment:

- **Reduce your stress:** Chronic stress and inflammation can harm the brain over time, contributing to neurodegenerative diseases. When you experience long-term stress, your body

continually releases stress hormones like cortisol. High levels of cortisol over time can damage parts of the brain involved in memory and learning.[8] Incorporate meditation, yoga, and journaling into your daily habits, and talk to a trusted counselor or clergy to lower your stress.
- **Keep learning:** Cognitive function is influenced by neuroplasticity, the brain's ability to form new neural connections, and declines without mental stimulation. Reading, working puzzles, learning new languages or dance steps, and playing musical instruments can keep the brain sharp.
- **Connect:** Social isolation is a risk factor for cognitive decline, with studies showing that staying socially engaged slows brain aging. Regular interactions with friends, family, and community members strengthen cognitive resilience and lower dementia risk.
- **Exercise for brain health:** Physical activity increases brain-derived neurotrophic factors, proteins essential for brain plasticity and learning.
- **Dietary interventions:** Foods rich in omega-3 fatty acids, antioxidants, and polyphenols (e.g., fish, berries, and green tea) protect the brain from oxidative damage.
- **Sleep:** Adequate sleep has a profound impact on brain health, promoting neurogenesis (new brain cell growth) and enhancing memory.

EMOTIONAL HEALTH: WHAT'S NORMAL AS YOU GROW OLDER?

The World Health Organization defines *emotional health* as the ability to cope with life's challenges, form meaningful relationships, manage emotions, and contribute to society.[9] This definition emphasizes not only the absence of mental illness but also the presence of positive mental states that enable individuals to realize their full potential, demonstrate resilience in the face of adversity, and actively participate in daily activities and their communities.

Research on emotional health and aging reveals that as they get older, people tend to have improved emotional regulation, meaning an increased ability to manage negative emotions and prioritize positive experiences. This "positivity effect" is a shift in attention toward positive stimuli, such as happy memories or favorable interpretations of events, that becomes more pronounced with age. Dr. Laura Carstensen's socioemotional selectivity theory argues that as people grow older and perceive their time as limited, they place greater importance on emotionally meaningful activities and relationships rather than novelty or career advancement. This shift fosters emotional well-being and life satisfaction in older adults. Compared to younger individuals, older adults report fewer negative emotions and a greater sense of emotional control. Even in stressful situations, older individuals are less likely to experience emotional volatility than younger adults, which has been attributed to their experience in managing interpersonal conflicts and emotional stressors over time.[10]

On the other hand, aging often brings major life transitions such as widowhood, retirement, chronic illness, and relocation. These transitions can increase social isolation, which, in turn, is linked to increased risks of depression and anxiety. Depression and anxiety in older adults is often underdiagnosed, as its symptoms—fatigue or reduced interest in activities—can be misinterpreted as "normal" signs of aging. Ensuring access to mental health care is critical for addressing these issues. Interventions like cognitive behavioral therapy and mindfulness-based stress reduction have proved effective in managing mental health challenges among older adults.

Emotional health plays a critical role in healthspan, contributing not only to individual well-being but also to cognitive and physical health. While it is normal to experience increased emotional stability and resilience, the risks of loneliness and depression remain significant challenges.

EMOTIONAL HEALTH: WHAT YOU CAN DO

Here's what you can do to maximize your emotional health:

- **Manage stress:** Mindfulness meditation, breathing exercises, and nature walks reduce stress and enhance emotional balance.
- **Cultivate positive emotions:** Practices like gratitude journaling and acts of kindness boost happiness and emotional well-being.
- **Stay connected:** Meaningful relationships with friends, family, or community groups are essential for maintaining emotional health.
- **Find purpose:** Engaging in activities that provide meaning—whether through work, volunteering, helping care for grandchildren, or creative expression—boosts well-being and longevity.
- **Seek support:** Therapy or support groups can help manage mental health challenges, ensuring emotional well-being throughout life.

––––––– JOY PRACTICE: –––––––
How Are Your Healthspan Habits?

Answer the following nine questions to take inventory of your current actions and attitudes related to healthspan. For each of the questions, rank yourself 1 to 5, with 1 being the worst and 5 being the best.

Do you move your body every day?

    Circle your self-rating: 1 2 3 4 5

Do you eat intentionally?

　　Circle your self-rating:　　1 2 3 4 5

Do you prioritize your sleep?

　　Circle your self-rating:　　1 2 3 4 5

Have you stopped/never started smoking?

　　Circle your self-rating:　　1 2 3 4 5

Do you avoid/limit alcohol consumption?

　　Circle your self-rating:　　1 2 3 4 5

Do you embrace growing older?

　　Circle your self-rating:　　1 2 3 4 5

Do you keep challenging yourself?

　　Circle your self-rating:　　1 2 3 4 5

Do you proactively cultivate friendships?

　　Circle your self-rating:　　1 2 3 4 5

Do you expect the best in your aging?

　　Circle your self-rating:　　1 2 3 4 5

Now add up your ratings from all nine categories. The maximum score is 45 points and the minimum score is 9 points.

INTERPRETATION:

- **40–45 points:** You are actively engaging in behaviors and mindsets that promote an extended healthspan. Keep it up!

- 21–39 points: There are significant opportunities for improvement—focus on areas where your scores are lower.
- 9–20 points: Your current habits and attitudes may be limiting your healthspan. Small changes in these areas can have a significant impact on your well-being.

Reflect on areas where improvement is needed and consider ways to enhance your physical, cognitive, and emotional well-being. Remember, even small adjustments—like increasing your daily movement or adopting a more optimistic outlook—can contribute meaningfully to a longer, healthier, and more fulfilling life.

HOW DOES JOYSPAN IMPROVE HEALTHSPAN?

A robust and growing body of research demonstrates that a longer *joyspan* can significantly impact *healthspan*. Joy is a biological and behavioral asset that extends healthspan by influencing multiple aspects of well-being. From lowering stress levels and enhancing immune function to encouraging healthy habits like exercise, sleep, and nutritious eating, joy has far-reaching effects on both mental and physical health.

Joyspan, cultivated through growth, connection, purpose, and adaptability, should be viewed as an essential component of preventive health care. By fostering joy and emotional well-being, you can proactively enhance your long life. Here are the biological mechanisms through which joyspan improves healthspan.

Cortisol Levels

Positive emotions, such as joy, help regulate the body's stress response by lowering cortisol levels. Chronic stress elevates cortisol, which can impair immune function, increase inflammation, and contribute to the development of chronic conditions like cardiovascular disease, diabetes, and depression. Joyful experiences promote relaxation and emotional balance, which reduce stress and protect long-term health.

Immune Function

Joy has been linked to stronger immune function. Positive emotional states trigger the release of neurotransmitters like serotonin and dopamine, which not only enhance mood but also improve immune response. A well-functioning immune system is essential for fending off infections and preventing the onset of chronic illnesses, thereby contributing directly to healthspan.

Cardiovascular Health

Studies show that people who maintain emotional well-being through joy and optimism are at lower risk for cardiovascular disease. Positive emotions lower blood pressure, improve heart rate variability, and decrease systemic inflammation, which reduces the likelihood of heart disease and stroke—two leading causes of mortality worldwide.

The Women's Health Initiative study examined morbidity, mortality, and chronic disease among ninety-five thousand women over an eight-year period. All of the women were free of cardiovascular disease and cancer at study entry. Participants with more positive emotions were less likely to develop coronary heart disease, were less likely to die from heart-related causes, and had lower total mortality due to all causes across the eight years of study. Positive emotional states were shown to be protective against stroke, carotid artery blockage, and rehospitalization.[11]

Physical Activity

People with higher levels of joy and positive emotions move more. Physical activity not only contributes to muscle strength and cardiovascular health but also supports mental well-being by releasing endorphins and other mood-enhancing chemicals. This feedback loop ensures that both physical and emotional health are maintained, creating a reinforcing cycle of healthy behavior.

Better Sleep Hygiene

People with more positive emotions are more likely to experience high-quality sleep, which is crucial for healthspan. Poor sleep is associated with increased risks of obesity, diabetes, and cognitive decline, while good sleep strengthens immunity, regulates metabolism, and enhances cognitive function.

Nutritious Diet and Healthy Choices

Positive emotional states encourage healthier eating patterns. Studies show that joyful individuals tend to consume more nutritious diets and avoid harmful behaviors such as excessive drinking or smoking. These habits prevent the onset of chronic diseases, further extending healthspan.

Connection

One of the strongest links between joyspan and healthspan is the role of relationships. The eighty-year Harvard Study of Adult Development found that individuals with fulfilling social connections experienced better mental and physical health over their lifetimes.[12] Strong relationships reduce loneliness—a major risk factor for mortality—and provide emotional support, helping people cope with challenges more effectively. The presence of joy in relationships also enhances mental resilience, which guards against depression and cognitive decline.

Resilience

Joy promotes emotional resilience, the ability to recover from stress and setbacks. Resilient individuals are less likely to develop stress-related illnesses and more capable of maintaining health through difficult times. This is critical for healthspan, as it reduces the risk of chronic diseases often associated with long-term stress, such as hypertension and depression.[13]

Healthspan is not everything; it's the power of small choices compounded over a lifetime. It is never too late, nor ever too soon to upgrade your physical, cognitive, and emotional health habits to lengthen your healthspan. Whether you start early or begin later, every choice matters. Starting where you are now, you can choose water over soda, an apple over Doritos, and movement over the couch. Today you can stretch, call a friend, take a walk, and schedule a doctor visit. None of this is revolutionary or complicated. Small choices, continued over your remaining lifetime, will shape your health.

In the next section we'll examine the interplay among the three aspects of longevity: lifespan, healthspan, and joyspan.

THE LONGEVITY PYRAMID: HOW LIFESPAN, HEALTHSPAN, AND JOYSPAN STACK UP

The Longevity Pyramid (see figure 6) offers a more comprehensive view of longevity and is a blueprint for understanding the multifaceted nature of healthy aging. It underscores the importance of moving beyond simply extending lifespan to ensuring that people enjoy long, healthy, and meaningful lives. Achieving joyspan requires intentional effort across all dimensions of health. Governments, health-care systems, families, and individuals must work together to foster environments where people are able to thrive at every stage of life.

FIGURE 6. The Longevity Pyramid

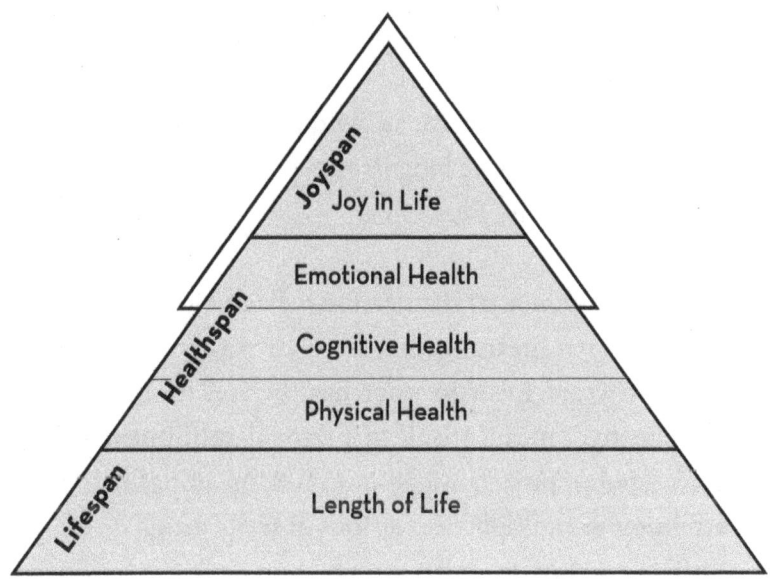

At the base of the pyramid lies **lifespan**, the total number of years a person lives. Lifespan provides the foundation upon which to build quality-of-life measures.

The second, narrower section of the pyramid is **healthspan**—the period of life spent in good health without significant disease or disability. Healthspan is divided into the three core dimensions: physical, cognitive, and emotional health. Together, these dimensions create a robust healthspan, ensuring not just survival but thriving across various aspects of life.

At the top of the pyramid is **joyspan**. It sits atop healthspan, representing the ultimate goal of living a contented and meaningful life. Joyspan refers to the portion of life characterized by continued growth, purpose, connection, and adaptation. It extends beyond health to include spiritual well-being, meaningful relationships, and the ability to find pleasure in everyday activities. Importantly, joyspan can exist even in the presence of health challenges, loss of loved ones, physical illness, and disability.

Achieving joyspan requires the integration of all levels—emotional stability, cognitive engagement, and physical health—to create a foundation on which joy and satisfaction can be built. Without these supports, it becomes harder for individuals to experience happiness consistently, even if they live long lives.

The pyramid structure illustrates:

1. **Interdependence of dimensions:** Each layer builds upon the previous one, meaning that lifespan without healthspan may result in years spent in poor health, and healthspan without joyspan may mean a lack of personal fulfillment. This interconnected approach suggests that a meaningful life requires attention to multiple dimensions of well-being.
2. **Shifting priorities with aging:** As people age, priorities tend to shift from simply extending life (lifespan), to maintaining independence and cognitive function (healthspan), and, ultimately, to finding joy and purpose (joyspan). This shift aligns with Dr. Laura Carstensen's socioemotional selectivity theory, which suggests that older adults prioritize emotionally meaningful goals as they age.
3. **Holistic aging strategies:** The diagram challenges the traditional focus on physical health by highlighting the importance of cognitive and emotional well-being. Policies and healthcare systems should adopt holistic aging strategies, supporting mental, emotional, and physical health equally.

Next let's consider how the elements of the Longevity Pyramid intersect using a Venn diagram of lifespan, healthspan, and joyspan. The **lifespan** circle (see figure 7) focuses on being alive: A long life is traditionally a desirable goal. At the middle left of the intersection, most people would agree that living a long, joyless life would be undesirable.

FIGURE 7. The Intersection Among Lifespan, Healthspan, and Joyspan

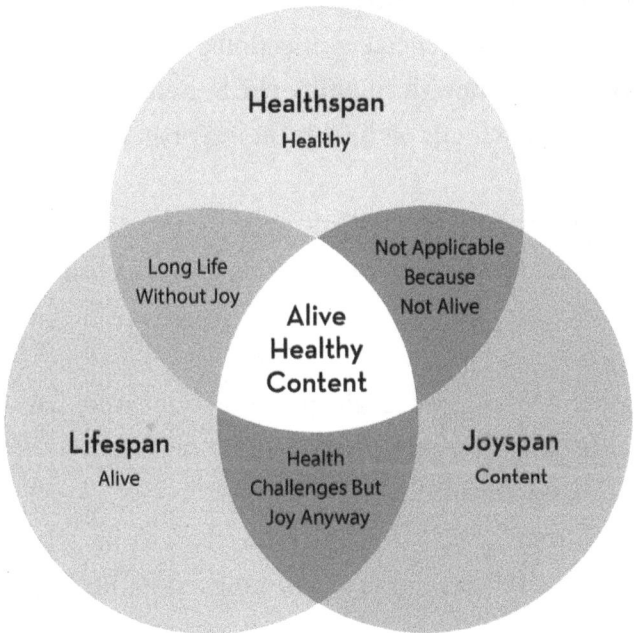

The **healthspan** circle addresses how long a person stays healthy, free from significant disease or disability. The intersection of healthspan and joyspan is "not applicable" because without lifespan (i.e., being alive), there can be no health or joy.

The **joyspan** circle emphasizes emotional well-being and fulfillment. As depicted in the lower center part of the intersection, a life with joy and purpose can make even the challenges of health problems more bearable.

At the center of the diagram, the optimal state is the intersection of being alive, healthy, and joyful. This intersection represents the goal: a life where all three dimensions—lifespan, healthspan, and joyspan—are in harmony. Achieving this state requires intentional effort across multiple areas:

1. **Maintaining physical and mental health** through proper nutrition, exercise, and preventive health care.
2. **Nurturing joy and purpose** by engaging in meaningful activities and fostering social connections.
3. **Living long enough to enjoy the benefits** of both health and joy through a focus on healthy aging practices.

This model emphasizes a holistic approach to well-being, suggesting that focusing too heavily on any one area can lead to an unbalanced life. For example:

- Lifespan without joy results in a long but empty life.
- Healthspan without joy leaves individuals physically well but emotionally unfulfilled.
- Joy without health demonstrates that while joy can persist through adversity, physical suffering limits life's opportunities and experiences.

The takeaway is that policies and personal strategies should aim to optimize all three dimensions: not just living long (lifespan) but living well (healthspan) and happily (joyspan). A life well-lived requires more than survival. It requires that we go beyond just treating illnesses (healthspan) or extending years (lifespan) and also focus upon optimal emotional health, living with joy, contentment, and purpose.

ATTITUDES AND ACTIONS FOR BETTER HEALTH

From the moment she became a mother thirty-one years ago, Elise always prioritized her family. Yes, she knew she could take better care of herself, but with all the demands of her four kids and their schedules, who had time? When she was fifty-nine, her husband, Pete, was diagnosed with Parkinson's disease. Witnessing his health challenges was a wake-up call. She realized that if she wanted to support him fully and be there for her family long-term, she needed to prioritize her own well-being.

Elise started small. She committed to a walk a day. She started to feel more energetic than she had in a decade and slowly added strength training and flexibility exercises on Mondays, Wednesdays, and Fridays. She noticed an improvement not only in her energy but also in her mood and focus.

Next, Elise decided to swap out processed foods for a balanced diet rich in fruits, vegetables, whole grains, and lean proteins. She adopted elements of the Mediterranean diet, using olive oil in her cooking and enjoying healthy fats from nuts and avocados. Not only did she feel more energized, but she also noticed her skin clearing up and her digestion improving.

One of the biggest challenges for Elise was adjusting her sleep habits. She knew all too well that sleep would help her brain stay sharp and her body stay resilient. She created a calming bedtime routine, avoiding screens and heavy meals in the evening. Sleeping still wasn't easy, but she started to find that her Apple Watch showed an increase in time slept. As another possible way to see if she could improve her sleep, Elise also decided to limit her alcohol intake. She had always enjoyed a glass of wine with dinner but wondered if reducing alcohol would help her feel better physically and mentally. It did. She switched to sparkling water with a slice of lemon at social gatherings and found she could enjoy herself just about as much without the alcohol.

Elise worked on looking at the aging process differently than she had in the past. She tried mindfulness exercises, focusing on self-acceptance, and called herself out when she found herself saying things like "I'm too old for that." She found that these practices reduced the strain she'd felt in "fighting aging," which helped her feel more at peace with herself and her life.

To keep her brain active, Elise made an effort to challenge herself regularly. She took up painting, started reading new genres of books, and even tried learning a new language. These activities kept her curious, engaged, and excited about personal growth. Elise made a point of reconnecting with old friends and actively seeking new connections, attending community events and joining a book club. These friendships brought joy and support, reinforcing the positive impact of social connections on her well-being (see figure 8).

Finally, Elise chose to expect the best in life. She started to notice how many negative and worried thoughts swirled around in her head. When

FIGURE 8. Joyspan Matrix in Action: Elise, Age 72

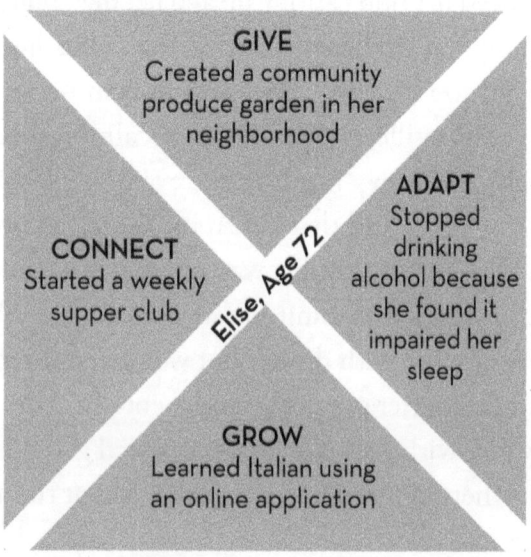

she noticed them, she would intentionally counter the worry with a reassuring thought. When her mind said, "My son's job seems unstable—what if he loses his job?" she would tell herself, "Don't borrow trouble. He has a job today, and today he is happy; if anything changes, he will be able to address it. He is thirty-two and capable." This shift not only helped her manage stress but also encouraged her to keep up with her healthy habits, knowing they would enhance her quality of life.

Through these changes, Elise transformed her life. By focusing on her healthspan and joyspan, she became more present, engaged, and resilient—ready to face the future with strength and positivity.

Like Elise, we can all make intentional improvements in our health habits. What one small change will you start with?

JOY PRACTICE:
One Small Change

Find a quiet place where you can write undisturbed for five minutes. Bring your journal or a piece of paper and allow yourself to answer these four questions freely and without judgment:

How well am I taking care of my body?
Am I challenging my brain through new learning and experiences?
How am I feeling emotionally?
What one small change will I start today to improve my healthspan?

For the last question, be specific in your answer! For example: "I will walk for fifteen minutes every morning; or I will call a friend or family member once a week; or I will read for twenty minutes before bed instead of scrolling on my phone." Close your entry by writing about how this small change will enhance your life and lead to other improvements.

JOYSPANNER: Dame Prue Leith

Born in 1940 in South Africa, Prue Leith is a restauranteur, broadcaster, writer and businesswoman. She was well known in culinary circles after founding Leith's School of Food and Wine in the 1970s, but became a household name after joining The Great British Bake Off as a judge in 2017 at age 77.

> **GROW:** In 2025, Prue appeared on TV show *The Masked Singer*. Despite thinking she couldn't sing, she took lessons and proved herself wrong. Speaking to a journalist about trying new things, she said: 'I'm a bit more reckless now. What's the worst that can happen?'
>
> **CONNECT:** Over the years, Prue has maintained connections to many friends and is close to her son Danny and adopted daughter Li-Da. In 2025, she stepped back from the celebrity edition of Bake Off to spend more time with her family.
>
> **ADAPT:** Prue's adaptability has seen her take on numerous challenges throughout her life. In her 80s she walked the catwalk at London Fashion Week, designed her own range of colourful glasses, and starred in a new cookery show with her husband.
>
> **GIVE:** Prue has campaigned for numerous causes, most recently in favour of bringing in laws to allow assisted dying in the UK.

PART II

What Strengthens Your Joyspan

PART II

What's Changing Your Lifespan

CHAPTER 4

Grow with Joy

Part 1 laid the foundation for how you think about your lifespan, healthspan, and joyspan. Now it's time to get down to business. Here you'll start the important work of strengthening your joyspan. You create your own joyspan through everyday choices that either help or hinder your ability to grow, connect, adapt, and give. This couldn't be more important because the quality of your life depends upon it. Let's look at how Betty maximized her joyspan and start at one of the lows of her long life.

When Betty was in her mid-fifties she walked into the kitchen to find her husband, John, slumped over the kitchen table in his plaid robe, his head in his hands. Wrapping her arms around his shoulders, she asked, "What is it, John?" He replied in a low voice gripped with great pain, "Bankruptcy."

As a child of the Great Depression, Betty had always been frugal. She was careful with money despite the material success John had enjoyed as a real estate developer. Now they were about to lose the business and their home. I was a junior in high school at the time and I, too, saw my usually joyful dad looking almost catatonic at the kitchen table. I even remember what he was wearing, a scratchy black-and-gray wool robe from Scotland. As if this news wasn't tough enough, the fall of his company also made the news, and it was in newspaper articles—we did not save these in our scrapbooks.

Although she'd been a first-grade teacher, Betty had stopped working to raise the kids, which was a long call of duty given that the youngest and oldest were sixteen years apart. We use the word "surprise" rather than "mistake," though both apply.

Betty was at one, of many, inflection points in the aging journey. We will all have these points, though with varying specifics—medical conditions, loss of a spouse, mobility or sensory impairment. At this inflection point, Betty went back to work.

"After thirty years off the job market, I felt like a fish out of water. It was a real stretch, an uncomfortably hard stretch to get back out there. My teaching credential was expired, and I needed to start earning quickly. I took stock of my skills to figure out what I could do, what I could offer." She drew upon one of the things she'd learned in the thirty years at home, home decorating. She went back to school to study interior design and was the oldest person in the room by two decades. While attending school, she offered her assistance to everyone she met—people at the market, the neighborhood, even at the vet. "It was awkward, hard, and I fumbled," she recalls. "But I grew, and I earned money for us to live on after we lost our home."

In the Joyspan Inventory in chapter 1, you responded to these two statements on growth:

1. *For me, life has been a continuous process of learning, changing, and growth.*

Strongly agree	Somewhat agree	Slightly agree	Neither agree nor disagree	Slightly disagree	Somewhat disagree	Strongly disagree
7	6	5	4	3	2	1

2. *I think it is important to have new experiences that challenge how I think about myself and the world.*

Strongly agree	Somewhat agree	Slightly agree	Neither agree nor disagree	Slightly disagree	Somewhat disagree	Strongly disagree
7	6	5	4	3	2	1

When you think about your continued growth right now, do you see yourself growing and expanding or are you feeling a bit stagnant or stuck? Regardless of where you find yourself now, you can increase your growth and improve your well-being.

What you can't afford to do is to give up on growth. "A significant proportion of the population has almost completely given up on learning. These people seldom, if ever engage in deliberate learning and see themselves as neither competent at it nor likely to enjoy it. The social and personal cost is enormous," writes researcher Dr. Seymour Papert. "Although negative self-images can be overcome, they are powerfully self-reinforcing. Deficiency becomes identity."[1] What self-limiting beliefs do you hold? Identify and banish thoughts like "I can't learn technology," or "I don't have a head for money," or "I'm not athletic." If you believe you can't learn new technology, you won't. The consequence of self-sabotage is failure, and each failure reinforces the original belief.

CONTINUED GROWTH MATTERS

Growth is the desire to explore, learn, and have new experiences. Lifelong growth is a key predictor of how we'll age. Without continued growth, we default to stagnation, defined as the lack of development or progress in physical health, mental and emotional well-being, social connections, and personal goals. Stagnation arises when you fail to find ways to contribute to the well-being of others and yourself. Stagnation leads to feelings of disconnection, boredom, and a sense of purposelessness.

Humans are driven to develop, acquire new skills, seek novelty, and expand. Adults who continue to grow have higher levels of life satisfaction, or what Dr. Carol Ryff describes as "psychological flourishing"—a sense of purpose and engagement.[2] Growth involves more than acquiring knowledge; it means being open to new encounters. Those who regularly engage in intellectual and emotional opportunities and challenges have lower rates of depression, anxiety, and cognitive decline.[3]

How do we continue to grow amid the pervasive messaging that aging is all decline? Research points to three critical factors: self-acceptance, curiosity, and humor.

SELF-ACCEPTANCE: THE FOUNDATION OF LIFELONG GROWTH

Self-acceptance is the ability to recognize and acknowledge all aspects of yourself—strengths and weaknesses—without self-criticism. Dr. Carl Rogers points to "the curious paradox, that when I accept myself just as I am, then I can change."[4] Self-acceptance leads to self-compassion, from which genuine growth can flourish.

People with greater self-acceptance are more resilient and have less anxiety and depression.[5] When you learn to accept yourself, you can pursue growth without feeling diminished by setbacks. This is especially important as we age. The goal is "identity resilience," the ability to see yourself less in terms of societal roles (such as career or family) and more in terms of internal qualities and personal values. This shift allows for a deeper level of self-acceptance and transcends surface appearance. As you move beyond the roles that defined you in youth, you have space to focus upon qualities like wisdom, patience, and compassion, embracing the richness of your experiences. You can celebrate inner gains rather than lamenting external losses.

Embracing Both Strengths and Weaknesses

Meaningful self-acceptance requires a balanced view of yourself. Regardless of how down you might feel right now, you do have strengths. And regardless of how well things are going, you make mistakes. All humans do. This integrated recognition prevents over-identification with either positive or negative traits. Self-acceptance based solely on strengths can be fragile, as it can lead you to deny or minimize your weaknesses, whereas a negative self-image can paralyze you from trying anything out of your comfort zone.

Buddhist monk and author Thich Nhất Hạnh offers this self-acceptance practice. When somebody compliments you, think: *You are only partly right, friend, in me there are good things. You should also know that in me there are also weaknesses and shortcomings.* In just the same way, when someone criticizes you, think: *You are only partly right, friend, in me there are weaknesses. You should also know that in me there are virtues and also talents.* With this practice you can see and accept yourself for who you really are.[6]

Cultivating Self-Acceptance

No one masters self-acceptance; it's an ongoing process that requires both awareness and effort. A proven way to increase self-acceptance is mindfulness. With all the talk about mindfulness these days, we've almost lost what it actually is. Mindfulness is just being present with yourself without judgment. When you take a moment to observe your thoughts and emotions, you create distance between yourself and your inner critic. Studies prove that mindfulness reduces self-criticism and enhances self-acceptance. Being mindful enables you to recognize that you are not defined by your thoughts or your emotions.

Another way to increase self-acceptance is a gratitude practice. This shifts your focus from what is lacking to what is already present and valuable. Brother David Steindl-Rast, a Benedictine monk, wrote, "The root of acceptance and joy is gratefulness."[7] By practicing gratitude, we can cultivate an appreciation for ourselves as we are, seeing our lives as sources of richness and growth rather than as incomplete or flawed.

Research consistently demonstrates that gratitude journaling enhances well-being and promotes self-acceptance as we grow older. Studies indicate that keeping a gratitude journal—regularly recording moments or aspects of life one is grateful for—can increase positive emotions, improve life satisfaction, and reduce symptoms of depression and anxiety.[8] Gratitude practices shift your focus toward the positive aspects of your life, which fosters contentment.

I gave my mom, Betty, a blank, lined journal and asked her to add one entry every day. Entry number 1 reads, "I am grateful for this blank book, it always feels so hopeful to start on a blank page. Entry 19, "Today I'm especially grateful for this warm cup of coffee as it's such a chilly morning." Entry 116, "Thank you God for being with me as I lay awake with a stomach ache last night." Entry 221, "I'm grateful for Elle who came and visited me today. She loves UCLA and that would make John so happy." She's numbered the entries and is currently at entry 681. I do the practice each day as well. It is never too soon to start the practice, and it is never too late. Writing what you are grateful for is helpful, and reviewing past entries is equally helpful. Bringing to mind what you are already grateful for helps you see other things throughout the day.

Psychologist Brené Brown's research highlights another effective way to cultivate your self-worth and self-acceptance: being vulnerable with others. Brown argues that by embracing vulnerability and showing up as we are, we allow others to see and accept us fully, which reinforces our own self-acceptance.[9] "You feel that way too?" is a path to self-acceptance. Knowing that everyone struggles with self-doubt reduces our own self-criticism.

Growing older also brings realizations about the folly of the being "special" myth. Betty put it this way: "In school I was never the smart one, the pretty one, the athletic one. But somehow, as I got older, I stopped feeling bad about not being 'the one' and felt better and better about just being ordinary." Ordinary is beautiful. You can finally be okay with all of you. You can free yourself from caring so much about others' opinions of you. As you grow older, you realize that people aren't thinking about you anyway. You can choose to treat yourself with kindness and compassion because you are inherently valuable. We all are.

THE BEST POSSIBLE FUTURE YOU

Is it possible to practice self-acceptance as we notice the external signs of aging? Wrinkles, age spots, thinning hair, muffin tops, turkey necks...can (and do) trigger insecurities, especially in a culture obsessed with youth. Is it possible to accept this version of ourselves? It is—and what's more, when you accept your aging self, it is possible to be beautiful all the way to the end. I know this to be true because I've seen it in thousands of people as they've aged. My mother, at age ninety-six, is one of many radiant older women and men around the globe.

Rather than striving to "preserve" a youthful appearance (which is impossible), these people have shifted to nurturing ageless qualities: kindness, curiosity, warmth, humor, generosity, strength, and resilience. When you feel at ease with yourself, your inner confidence shines through, creating a presence that transcends physical appearance. This magnetic energy draws people to you not for how you look, but for how you make them feel. Those who radiate such timeless beauty as they age have accepted themselves.

> "The less attention you pay to how others perceive you, the more energy you put into what matters to you *intrinsically*, the more you flourish at what you genuinely care about, the more your aesthetics improve, the better you are perceived."
>
> —Isabel Hazan, blogger

Dr. Laura King, a professor at the University of Missouri, Columbia, created an experiment for people of all ages. In her study, participants were asked to write about their best possible future self for twenty minutes daily over several consecutive days. The findings revealed significant increases in overall well-being and optimism with effects that lasted even after the exercise ended. King noted that envisioning an ideal future self helped individuals clarify their goals, feel more hopeful, and feel more control over their lives.* Further research has confirmed the exercise's benefits across different demographics, suggesting its broad applicability. Those who participated reported an enhanced sense of purpose and motivation, likely because focusing on an ideal future self can reduce rumination on current or past difficulties.† King's work on this exercise has been instrumental in establishing it as a key tool in positive psychology, with a clear impact on emotional resilience and life satisfaction.

---

* Laura A. King, "The Health Benefits of Writing About Life Goals," *Personality and Social Psychology Bulletin* 27, no. 7 (2001): 798–807.

† Laura A. King, "Intervention for Enhancing Subjective Well-Being: Can We Make People Happier and Should We?," in *The Science of Subjective Well-Being*, ed. Michael Eid and Randy J. Larsen (Guilford Press, 2008), 431–48.

———— JOY PRACTICE: ————
The Best Possible Future You

This exercise helps you cultivate self-acceptance as you navigate the exterior signs of aging. You can embrace the aging process with grace, authenticity, and confidence by envisioning the future you. Once you envision the kind of older person you'd like to be, you will consciously (and unconsciously) cultivate those characteristics.

- **Step 1. List enduring qualities:** Take a moment to write down qualities you admire that go beyond physical appearance. These could include kindness, resilience, humor, generosity, warmth, and strength. Think about how people you admire—public or private figures—embody these qualities. Consider what you appreciate about them and how their presence makes you feel. Next, circle the qualities that feel most important to you personally. Reflect on why these qualities matter and how they make others beautiful, regardless of age.
- **Step 2. Write about the future you:** Write about a future self that embodies the qualities you listed in the first step. Be as specific and aspirational as possible—really go for it. Write about how radiant, kind, funny, joyful, energetic, and thoughtful (or whatever you value) you are and how you make people feel in your presence.
- **Step 3. Set your intention:** Write two actions you will take to cultivate the qualities you've chosen. For example, if you want to embody authenticity, you might commit to allowing yourself to be vulnerable with yourself and others. If you admire resilience, think about how you can approach life's challenges with greater acceptance. Choose a phrase or mantra to remind yourself of your commitment, such as "My authenticity (or resilience or kindness, etc.) makes me radiant."

Completing this exercise will clarify what "success" in longevity means to you. You won't be trying to *appear* a certain way, you will be seeking to *embody* your chosen traits. So focus on growing into the best version of yourself internally. How you look to others will take care of itself.

CURIOSITY: THE GROWTH CATALYST

Curiosity—the desire to seek new knowledge—plays a fundamental role throughout life. Curiosity fosters continued intellectual, emotional, and spiritual growth. Curiosity is a willingness to ask questions, to try new or unfamiliar experiences. Rather than external rewards or goals, curiosity is driven by interest and the joy of discovery.

Researchers have identified two main types of curiosity: *epistemic*, which is acquiring new information; and *perceptual*, which involves sensory exploration and seeking novelty. Both forms of curiosity play a crucial role in growth and well-being in later life.

As you age, engaging in curiosity-driven activities promotes neuroplasticity, which is the brain's ability to reorganize itself by forming new neural connections. Great curiosity improves memory retention, particularly in older adults, suggesting that curiosity is not only an outcome of growth but also a catalyst for it. Research shows that people who remain curious are better able to navigate life transitions, adapt to new circumstances, and maintain a positive outlook.[10] This flexibility contributes to sustained intellectual, emotional, and spiritual growth because curious individuals remain open to new possibilities and to expand their understanding.

Curiosity and Intellectual Growth

You are never too old and it is never too late to become curious. Intellectual growth comes not only from education, but also from reading, asking questions, and having new experiences. Learning is widely recognized as a protective factor against cognitive decline. Engaging in intellectually stimulating activities forms new neural connections, bolsters memory retention, and supports overall mental acuity. Cognitive neuroscience shows that learning stimulates the production of brain-derived neurotrophic factors, proteins that support the growth and survival of neurons. This stimulation is particularly effective in the hippocampus, a brain region vital for memory and learning.

Several longitudinal studies illustrate the benefits of lifelong learning for cognitive health. The Advanced Cognitive Training for Independent and Vital Elderly (ACTIVE) study, a landmark trial in cognitive aging, found that individuals who engaged in regular cognitive training showed improvements in memory, reasoning, and processing speed that lasted up to five years postintervention.[11] Another study from the American Academy of Neurology suggests that people who participate in intellectually engaging activities, such as reading, writing, or puzzles, exhibit a significantly slower rate of cognitive decline compared to those who are less active mentally.[12]

Intellectual curiosity is the desire to learn or understand something unfamiliar. Contrary to the outdated notion that curiosity diminishes with age, psychological research shows that curiosity can be cultivated at any stage of life and remaining curious can foster a sense of purpose and contribute to overall life satisfaction.[13] Even after controlling for all confounding factors, older adults with high levels of curiosity perform better in memory performance and problem-solving tasks compared to those with lower curiosity levels.[14] What are you curious about? Do you have an interest in learning a new language? Going somewhere new? Teaching someone something?

There are numerous ways to integrate learning into your life. Universities and organizations like the University of the Third Age (U3A) provide programs tailored to adults, allowing you to pursue courses in anything you are curious about. There are also sources of self-directed learning, such as online courses, podcasts, virtual museum tours, live-streamed lectures, and language-learning apps. A good approach is to start with one in-person learning opportunity (community center, university) and one technology-based learning opportunity (online) to see which you enjoy the most. Many people find they love both! My friend Jan took a course and liked it so much that she ended up teaching it the following semester. She's been teaching the course for six years now and recently mused, "Who knew I'd be teaching a course in interior design at eighty-three, but here I am, and my class size grows every semester!"

Intellectual curiosity, often underestimated in later years, is a catalyst for growth. Cultivating your curiosity boosts your brain and helps you discover, or rediscover, your passion.

> At age ninety-five, Nola Ochs graduated from Fort Hays State University in Kansas after earning a general studies degree with an emphasis in history. Not content to stop there, she completed a master's degree in liberal studies at ninety-eight, proving that age is no barrier to academic achievement. On her curiosity and love for learning, Nola remarked, "I don't dwell on my age. I just live and do what I can and enjoy life."

Curiosity and Emotional Growth

Curiosity also drives emotional growth, enhancing empathy and interpersonal connections. Adults who are curious about the perspectives and experiences of others are more likely to build meaningful relationships, contributing to their emotional growth and sense of belonging.[15] Emotional curiosity enhances both personal and relational aspects of emotional well-being. Curiosity enables people to approach difficult emotions with openness rather than avoidance.

Curiosity-driven exploration is helpful as you navigate life changes such as retirement, loss of a loved one, and physical limitations. Growing older can be hard, but emotional curiosity helps.

Retirement left Julia with unstructured time, and she grappled with feeling down. "I just felt blah, like, what's the point now?" Julia sighed. She'd always been practical and grounded, but with her routines disrupted, she felt unmoored and if she was honest, pretty awful. One day, during a quiet afternoon at home, Julia viewed her feelings with curiosity rather than trying to push them down. In examining how she felt with objectivity, she realized that her sense of loneliness stemmed not only from the physical absence of colleagues but also from a deeper longing for meaning. Writing openly and honestly, Julia journaled about her unspoken fears about the future, about losing her identity, her health, her independence. By examining the fears rather than avoiding them, she felt a sense of relief that surprised her. Facing her fears head-on not only helped her but also enabled Julia to help her friends, who she learned were also grappling with unacknowledged fears around growing older.

Curiosity and Spiritual Growth

As you face profound transitions such as the loss of a loved one or changes in health, curiosity can fuel spiritual growth. You might seek answers to questions that may have lingered throughout life: Am I living my life well? How am I connected to others, to a higher power, and to the universe? Curiosity can motivate you to study spiritual practices, philosophies, and religious teachings. Through this process, you not only learn but also cultivate inner peace, acceptance, and a broader perspective.

I was blessed to know a woman named Maria. She had led a full life as a mother, a teacher, and an active community member. In her late eighties, she began to feel a deep sense of loss as friends and family members passed away. Her world grew smaller, and she found herself questioning her purpose and legacy.

Instead of withdrawing into sadness, though, Maria's curiosity led her on an unexpected spiritual journey. She'd been a Catholic all her life, and her faith meant a great deal to her. Without giving up Catholicism, she began reading books on other religious and spiritual traditions, from Buddhism to Sufism.

Maria's curiosity brought her to a meditation group at our community center. Initially hesitant, she joined the group with an open mind and a spirit of exploration. She soon found solace and connection, learning to sit in silence and reflect on life's deeper mysteries. The practice of meditation helped her come to terms with her losses and accept her own mortality. She described this period as a "quiet awakening," in which she felt a renewed sense of peace, purpose, and connection to God.

FIGURE 9. Joyspan Matrix in Action: Maria, Age 72

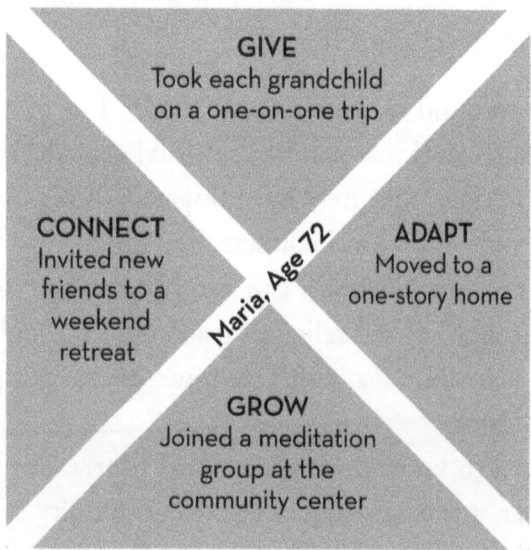

Exploring spiritual questions may lead you to grapple with the realities of aging and mortality with inquisitiveness. Spiritual curiosity encourages the view that life is an ongoing process, and that each stage has its own wisdom to offer.

In Maria's case, her curiosity allowed her to approach aging with more wonder. She found comfort in the idea that her spirit was part of something larger than herself, connected to others and to the cosmos. Spiritual growth often continues as long as you remain curious about it.

You have seen how curiosity is essential to continued intellectual development, emotional resilience, and spiritual depth. By nurturing curiosity, you build capacity for growth. Knowledge, understanding, and personal development are lifelong endeavors (see figure 9).

—— JOY PRACTICE: ——
I'm Curious About...

This exercise is a springboard for cultivating your curiosity. Use the list below to check off anything that intrigues you. If you don't see something listed, add it in the blank spots at the bottom. Next, put a star next to each of your top five.

NATURE

- ☐ Camping/backpacking
- ☐ Hiking/trail work
- ☐ Gardening
- ☐ Nature photography
- ☐ Bird-watching
- ☐ Conservation

CREATIVITY

- ☐ Painting or drawing
- ☐ Pottery or ceramics classes
- ☐ Writing (fiction, poetry, nonfiction, memoir)

- ☐ Musical instruments
- ☐ Dance (swing, ballroom, ballet, jazz, tap, modern)
- ☐ Choir or an a cappella group
- ☐ Knitting, crochet, needlepoint
- ☐ Bookmaking/scrapbooking
- ☐ Photography

Fitness

- ☐ Yoga
- ☐ Pilates
- ☐ Tai chi
- ☐ Running
- ☐ Weight lifting
- ☐ Pickleball
- ☐ Swimming
- ☐ Golf
- ☐ Surfing and stand-up paddleboarding
- ☐ Walking
- ☐ Canoeing and kayaking
- ☐ Skiing, snowboarding, snowshoeing

Learning

- ☐ Book club
- ☐ History class
- ☐ Language class
- ☐ Art class
- ☐ Cooking class
- ☐ Wine course
- ☐ Genealogy
- ☐ Piano lessons
- ☐ Dance class
- ☐ Public speaking
- ☐ Boating

Community Engagement

- ☐ Tutoring youth
- ☐ Fostering children
- ☐ Serving in soup kitchens
- ☐ Faith community involvement
- ☐ Volunteering in skilled nursing facility
- ☐ Hospice volunteer
- ☐ Civic club member

Home

- ☐ Interior design projects
- ☐ Upscaling furniture
- ☐ Collecting art
- ☐ Antiquing
- ☐ Flipping houses

Personal Growth

- ☐ Gratitude journaling
- ☐ Wellness retreats
- ☐ Vision boards
- ☐ Faith practices
- ☐ Meditation and prayer
- ☐ Creating a new relationship
- ☐ Nurture an existing relationship

Travel and Adventure

- ☐ Solo travel
- ☐ Group travel
- ☐ Road trips to explore nearby towns
- ☐ Sailing or motorboating
- ☐ Boat cruises
- ☐ National parks
- ☐ Historic sites
- ☐ Cycling trips
- ☐ Voluntourism

Finance

- ☐ Managing investments
- ☐ Day-trading
- ☐ Entrepreneurship
- ☐ Financial planning for retirement
- ☐ Consulting

Technology and Digital Skills

- ☐ Social media
- ☐ Video editing classes
- ☐ Digital scrapbooking
- ☐ Online gaming
- ☐ Virtual reality

PETS AND ANIMAL COMPANIONS

- ☐ Fostering pets
- ☐ Dog-walking group
- ☐ Volunteering at animal shelters
- ☐ Learning pet photography

SUSTAINABLE LIVING

- ☐ Practicing eco-friendly habits and reducing waste
- ☐ Growing a vegetable or herb garden at home
- ☐ Supporting local or organic farmers and markets
- ☐ Vintage fashion and thrifting
- ☐ Environmental conservation

OTHER (ADD YOUR IDEAS HERE)

_____

_____

Now that you've sparked your curiosity, you can set your "curiosity goals." Unlike traditional goals, which often focus on specific achievements, curiosity-oriented goals are designed to encourage exploration and learning. For instance, you might set a goal to read a book on a topic you know little about, attend a lecture on a new subject, or explore a new hobby each month. Curiosity-oriented goals can be flexible and open-ended, allowing you to adapt your interests as they grow.

HUMOR IS NO LAUGHING MATTER

Kids laugh all the time—three hundred times a day on average. A Gallup poll of 1.4 million respondents across 166 countries reveals, however, that laughter declines sharply around age twenty-three and continues to dip into middle age. By the age of forty, the average person laughs only three hundred times every 2.5 months, translating to approximately four laughs a day. But the great news is that the laughing curve goes up again after age ninety—due to extended longevity, enhanced health, and, most importantly, greater joy.[16] Humor is essential for continued growth because humor promotes health, coping, and the willingness to try new things. In the rest of this chapter, I'll explore the science behind the laughter curve, discuss the critical role humor plays in continued growth, and suggest how you can start laughing more today.

> "Give me a soul that knows not boredom, grumblings, sighs and laments, nor excess of stress, because of that obstructing thing called 'I.' Grant me, O Lord, a sense of good humor. Allow me the grace to be able to take a joke, to discover in life a bit of joy, and to be able to share it with others."
> —*Thomas More, 1498*

Humor and Your Physical Health

Humor impacts physical health through laughter, which releases endorphins and reduces markers of inflammation, the precursor to most chronic diseases. Laughter improves blood flow and lowers blood pressure. Laughter has effects on the cardiovascular system similar to those of aerobic exercise, making it a valuable addition to a heart-healthy lifestyle. Laughter strengthens the immune system by reducing the stress hormone cortisol, which can weaken immune system response.[17]

A study published in *Psychology and Aging* found that adults who regularly engaged in humor-based activities performed better on memory and cognition tests. Adults who use humor experience increased cognitive flexibility and problem-solving abilities.[18] If you don't feel that you're laughing much, do not despair. When it comes to laughter, you can always level up.

I met Margaret when she was seventy-nine because she had been struggling to retrieve words. A retired accountant, she liked precision and order. She had little patience for jokes or humor. Though a neuropsychological evaluation did not find cognitive impairment, Margaret still was worried sick. We brainstormed ideas until landing on one that most intrigued (and scared) Margaret—a laughter yoga session at the community center. A laughter yoga class is led by a teacher who instructs participants in traditional stretches and poses in yoga and also incorporates a series of exercises that ask participants to say "Ha" a number of times while posing. As the "Ha's" accumulate, laughing ensues, often with resulting hilarity. At first, Margaret felt out of place, her old habits of reserve and control surfacing as everyone around her laughed and played. As other students let out their "ha-ha's," she began to let go. Over the next few weeks, she returned to the classes and started pushing herself to explore humor in other areas of her life as well. She started watching comedy shows, learning some simple jokes to share with her grandkids, and even read books on the benefits of humor. An accountant's approach! To her surprise, laughter and humor felt good—almost like a mental release she hadn't known she needed.

Within a few months, Margaret felt more alert, found herself recalling information more easily—even her problem-solving skills seemed sharper. Inspired, Margaret read a study about how humor activates the brain's reward centers, releasing dopamine and promoting cognitive flexibility. She realized that laughter was a mental exercise, helping her stay sharp and engaged with the world.

Humor as a Life Raft

In life, things sometimes go wrong. *Saturday Night Live* comedian Gilda Radner, in her thirties at the time, was having a hard time getting pregnant. After months of dismissing bloating and cramping, Radner was diagnosed with stage 4 ovarian cancer. In her memoir, *It's Always Something*, she describes her illness with raw honesty and humor. The book encourages others to find moments of joy and resilience in their own struggles.

According to her husband, actor Gene Wilder, humor allowed Gilda to maintain her identity and spirit despite her cancer. While enduring great physical pain and emotional turmoil, Radner's humor was a form of resistance—a way of asserting her humanity in the face of a disease that could otherwise strip it away.

Even for those of us who are not comedians, humor serves as a coping mechanism for navigating life when things go wrong. Research reveals that humor reduces anxiety and depression and increases resilience.[19] Humor allows us to view challenges from a different perspective, making problems more relatable and perhaps more manageable.

> "Comedy is about what goes wrong with the world—people laugh because something is too big, or too small, or too much, or not enough."
> —*Gilda Radner, comedian*

Humor Helps You Try New Things

My dad was funny. He was always sharing jokes and a quick laugh at himself and things around him. I suspect his humor was in response to his hard childhood. His mother left his father and their three sons, ages seven, six, and four at the time. My father was the youngest and has few memories of his mom, but he does remember the slap in the face she gave him. My grandfather had to put the three boys in a place called the "Busy Bee" boarding school. "It wasn't the fancy kind of boarding school; it was the kind where kids got dropped off by people who drove away fast," my dad recalls. "Yeah, there were a lot of tears there."

As my dad grew up, moments of laughter created a welcome break from the grind and also bolstered him to put himself out there and try new things. He had never known anyone who'd attended college. One day when he was working at a shoe store, he was sliding a shoe onto the foot of a young man. "The fellow said he was getting new sneakers to start at UCLA in the fall. We got to talking and I peppered him with questions on how a guy gets to go to college. That fellow told me just what he did, and you know what? I followed it to the letter. I didn't have two dimes to rub together, but at that time you only needed a C grade point average, so I went for it," he explained with a grin. He got in, worked three jobs, graduated, and enjoyed a fulfilling career. My dad's humor bolstered him to try new things all life long. My mother remarked, "I was the straight man, to John's sense of humor. As I grew older, I realized that I could choose to laugh and now I do it every day. Humor has made me bolder, too! If these walls could talk, they'd tell of an old woman who not only talks to herself but laughs out loud at what she says."

How to Cultivate Humor

Can you become funnier and learn to laugh more on a daily basis? Yes! Known for his sharp wit, Archbishop Desmond Tutu advised, "I don't think I woke up and presto I was funny. I think it is something that you can cultivate. Like anything else, it is a skill. The easiest place to start is laughing at yourself. If you start looking for the humor in life, you will find it. It makes everything easier including your ability to accept others and accept all that life will bring."[20]

> "A sense of humor is the pole that adds balance to our steps as we walk the tightrope of life."
> —Mahatma Gandhi

Humor can be practiced and improved like any other interpersonal skill. You develop humor by watching funny movies and TV shows, reading funny books, watching comedians, engaging in playful activities, telling jokes, and observing the humorous styles of others.

Want to be funnier? Hang out with people who make you laugh. People learn behaviors by observing and imitating others. Humor matters and can be cultivated through practice, reflection, and intentional activities. Humor training can increase an individual's ability to handle stress and improve emotional resilience. Many psychologists encourage clients to reframe negative thoughts with a humorous perspective, which can increase their ability to find humor in challenging situations. This reframing approach has been found to improve mood and reduce anxiety.[21]

JOY PRACTICE:
It's Funny, Really

Make a habit of finding at least one thing to laugh about each day. Here's a list to get you started:

- Laugh at your next mistake. In fact, make it a belly laugh and try talking to yourself out loud in a lighthearted way. If you are alone, great. If not, you are likely to make others laugh, which is a good thing, too.

- Ask around for recommendations of funny movies or TV series. Laugh out loud as you watch them.
- Call someone who makes you laugh. Even if you haven't spoken in years, track them down and reconnect.
- Find an in-person or online "laughter yoga class." This practice combines intentional laughter with breathing exercises and has been found to improve mood and reduce stress.
- When you are at the supermarket, seek moments of connection over things that strike you as funny: the shape of a particular eggplant!
- Watch a stand-up comedian special on TV or go to a comedy club.
- Learn some jokes and then practice telling them to anyone who will listen, from your grandchildren to your doctor. Here's one to get you started: "What is the difference between a dirty bus stop and a lobster with chest implants? One is a crusty bus station and one is a busty crustacean." Laugh at your own joke, especially if no one else is.

GROWTH VIA BELLY FLOP

I learned about growth via a loud and public belly flop. With my seven-year-old legs shaking, I climbed up the tall ladder of the (very) high dive at the community pool. I put my spindly arms straight up by my ears and clasped them together. Teeth chattering, I edged to the end and clenched my toes over the edge. After too long, I gave it a little bounce and launched. The result was not a dive; it was a loud, epic bellyflop. It felt like an openhanded belly smack from King Kong.

Gasping for breath, I started crying and struggled to the edge of the pool. Observers let out audible "oooofs" and stifled chuckles. I don't blame them; my belly was a bright red from the smacking and my face matched from embarrassment. Betty and John saw the flop and I suspect they were not overly surprised—what their youngest had in enthusiasm she lacked in athleticism. My parents suggested I go back up and try it again.

"You can do it!" Their dorky cheerleading was as embarrassing as the belly smacking itself. Horrified, I narrowed my eyes and silently implored them to seriously stop. They did not. To stop this awful scene, I got back up on the death trap and did the stupid dive. That night, my mom pulled out a charm from her jewelry box that read "true grit." The ability to find courage and resolve in hard circumstances. The reason she had such a charm was that my father had given it to her after they'd gone through a rough economic patch.

Not unlike the belly flop, lifelong personal growth will require you to pick yourself up, dust yourself off, and dive back in. It is in fact never too late to put in the work to remain vital throughout your life. The effort you invest in health habits (moving, eating real food, sleeping, connecting) pays off handsomely in quality of later life. In thinking about your continued personal growth, consider these juicy questions:

- Am I using my life well?
- Have I experienced all the things I want to experience?
- Am I doing what I love to do?
- Am I helping others?
- Who will be at my memorial service and what will they say?

KEEP GROWING

This chapter explored the first element: growth. You maximize this element with intentional effort and joy practices in self-acceptance, curiosity, and humor. What happens when you keep growing?

You will improve your cognitive health: Growth, particularly intellectual and creative growth, keeps the mind active, which is essential for cognitive health. Engaging in activities that challenge the brain—such as learning a new language, exploring hobbies, or solving problems—enhances memory ability and cognitive function. Studies show that cognitive stimulation helps delay mental decline, allowing people to remain sharp and independent longer, which greatly enhances their quality of life.

You will experience a sense of accomplishment: Continuously setting and achieving personal goals, no matter how small, brings a sense of pride and accomplishment. This sense of progress is deeply satisfying and reinforces self-worth and confidence. Feeling capable and accomplished fosters a positive self-image, which can counteract the negative stereotypes around aging and contribute to a joyful and empowered experience of growing older.

You will enjoy greater emotional resilience and adaptability: Growth promotes emotional resilience, helping people approach life's challenges with a positive, adaptable mindset. By continuously seeking to learn and improve, individuals build skills for coping with losses, health issues, and other challenges that often come with aging. This growth-oriented mindset allows older adults to view setbacks not as threats to happiness but as opportunities for learning and strengthening resilience, which boosts long-term well-being.

You will strengthen your relationships: Growth in emotional intelligence can enhance empathy, communication, and relationship-building skills. As people grow, they often become more understanding and patient, which serves to strengthen connections with family, friends, and the community. These meaningful connections provide emotional support and companionship, both of which are crucial to maintaining happiness as people age.

You will have an impact: When you focus on your growth, you are likely to inspire others. Often, you never even know about the impact you have, but that doesn't make it any less meaningful.

Keep your growth tank full to remain vibrant, connected, and purpose-driven, transforming aging from something to fear into an opportunity for deeper joy, wisdom, and self-fulfillment. In the next chapter we'll explore the second tank of joyspan, connection.

JOYSPANNER: Gyles Brandreth

Born in 1948, Gyles Brandreth is a British broadcaster, writer and former politician.

> **GROW:** Gyles is always finding new ways to share his passions with others. As well as launching the Poetry Together project with HRH Queen Camilla in 2019, he has taken to podcasting and even relaunched his own brand of knitwear to reach a new audience.
>
> **CONNECT:** After the Covid-19 pandemic, Gyles has spoken out about how important community and connection are for wellbeing, especially after spending so much time alone in lockdown.
>
> **ADAPT:** In his book *The 7 Secrets of Happiness* Gyles says that embracing change is one of the keys to being joyful. A true joyspanner!
>
> **GIVE:** Gyles has publicly supported a great number of charities over his lifetime, including Comic Relief,

Arthritis Research and Water Aid. Most recently, in 2023, he became the first official patron for Schoolreaders, a charity providing primary schools with dedicated volunteers to support children's reading on a one-to-one basis.

CHAPTER 5

Connect to Joy

Byron was one of my father's closest friends. Nearly a full head taller than my father, Byron was a handsome giant who lit up the room. Between my dad's renowned humor and Byron's smile, the two friends were quite a pair. I can still picture Byron leaning over my dad's hospital bed with his big hand atop my dad's hand the week he died. My dad died when he was eighty-three, and Byron died just recently at ninety years old. My mother and I attended Byron's celebration of life luncheon. Hundreds of his friends attended and when the opportunity for impromptu speeches arose, person after person stood up and took a turn. Nearly everyone said that Byron was one of their closest friends. In their words I heard clues about what it takes to form meaningful connections. Each person talked about how Byron called them regularly, for no other reason than to hear how they were. He was the one who instigated plans to get together, and posted a list of birthdays, anniversaries, dates of people's passing, and other memorable days on his wall. He used this list to remind himself to call or send people a message or note on those days. When someone went into the hospital, it was Byron by their bedside.

Byron wasn't just lucky; he took the time, thought, and energy it required to become a cherished friend. He gave freely. He did not fall prey to damaging thoughts like, "Why am I the one who always calls to make plans?" Toward the end of his life, he continued his outreach from a wheelchair and while juggling doctor appointments, hospitalizations, and pain. Byron poured himself into connection.

> "We cannot live only for ourselves. A thousand fibers connect us with our fellow men; and among those fibers, as sympathetic threads, our actions run as causes, and they come back to us as effects."
> —Herman Melville, author

The second element of joyspan is Connect. **Connection** refers to meaningful bonds with others and is created by fostering relationships that provide support, companionship, and belonging. Fortunately, you can actively nurture connection if: (1) you know how; and (2) you are willing to make some effort. It doesn't happen by chance; you'll need to consciously foster and create bonds.

In this chapter I'll explain why connections are critical to joyspan; how to stay connected to family (biological and chosen) and friends; how to know if you are lonely; how to take inventory of your current connections; and how to find new friends.

> "The best thing I've done is to make new friends along the way. What's surprised me is how much sweeter the friendships are now. There is more depth in our connection. We look out for each other. We need each other."
> —Betty, age ninety-six

YOUR JOYSPAN NEEDS QUALITY CONNECTIONS

Quality connections are crucial for joyspan because humans are social beings. Whether you are an introvert or an extrovert, you are hardwired for connection—it's embedded in your biology. Connections are a powerful predictor of both mental and physical health, and having healthy relationships has been shown to reduce stress, boost the immune system, lower blood pressure, reduce inflammation, and help stave off loneliness, depression, and slow cognitive decline. Relationships stimulate the release of hormones like oxytocin and endorphins, which promote feelings of happiness and reduce stress. Without regular, meaningful interactions, we miss out on these benefits, making it harder to feel energized, resilient, and positive as we grow older.

The data on human connection is compelling. Your social connections are as significant a predictor of longevity as factors like diet, exercise, and even smoking. In fact, a lack of social connection does greater harm to health than obesity and high blood pressure. Dr. Julianne Holt-Lunstad analyzed 148 epidemiological studies on the predictors of mortality. Combined, the studies include data on more than three hundred thousand patients. The studies examined the role of physical factors such as alcohol, weight, smoking, exercise, prescribed and recreational drugs, vaccines, and air pollution. Research also looked at social factors including number and quality of friendships, participation in social activities, partner status, isolation, and feelings of loneliness. The findings were clear and astounding. It was the social measures that best predicted whether a patient survived a stroke or a heart attack. Those who had more frequent social interaction and felt integrated into a community or network increased their chances of surviving by *50 percent*![1]

Psychologists define a quality connection as being seen, heard, and valued by another human. You might experience it in a family member's knowing gaze; a shared laugh with someone when you both realize you thought you were "the only one who..."; the shared pleasure of a colorful sunset. Moments of quality connection bring color and depth to our days, reminding us that we're part of something greater than ourselves.

In the second half of life, connection can include relationships with neighbors, relatives, longtime friends, new friends, coworkers, and those we love but haven't seen for a long time, as well as chance encounters—those we help, those who help us, and other people we meet. As we grow older, connection becomes *more* essential, not less. In times of adversity or loss, connections provide a buffer, allowing us to recover and continue with a renewed or new purpose. Connection transforms the experience of aging from a solitary to a shared journey, where moments of joy are multiplied and burdens are lightened.

How do you make sure you are connected? The three critical elements of connection in the joyspan model are existing connections, new connections, and interdependence. Let's start with interdependence.

THE MYTH OF INDEPENDENCE

One of the myths about growing older is that you must maintain your independence. The reality is that you were never independent to begin with. In childhood, you depended upon parents, siblings, teachers, and friends. As you grew, there was a developmental imperative to try to assert your independence, a necessary, appropriate developmental progression.

> "In the progress of personality, first comes declaration of independence, then a recognition of interdependence."
>
> *—Henry Van Dyke, former US ambassador to the Netherlands*

In contemporary society, independence is often upheld as a marker of success and self-worth. People are encouraged to "stand on their own two feet," to be "self-made," and to pursue individual goals with minimal reliance on others. Yet the idea of complete independence—of existing and succeeding entirely on one's own—is a myth. This myth can be isolating and even damaging, as it leads you to undervalue relationships, avoid seeking help, and feel inadequate when you inevitably need support.

We were designed for connection, and we are harmed by loneliness. According to the American Psychiatric Association's latest poll, released in late January 2024, one in three people in America feels lonely every week, and 10 percent feel lonely every single day.[2] Loneliness is a universal feeling, and it often has to do with feeling not understood. Once you make that connection with other people—that they feel or have felt the same—it feels like a weight is taken off your shoulders.

> "I struggled over the years with depression, anxiety, and loneliness. It's not just a feeling that I get when I'm alone. I also feel lonely sometimes sitting right next to my husband and sometimes I get lonely in a group of people."
> —*Kate, age seventy-eight*

Embracing interdependence allows people to lean on one another during tough times, building a supportive network that fosters mental and emotional well-being. When we contribute to the well-being of others, we experience a sense of accomplishment and purpose that goes beyond individual success. Interconnectedness not only fulfills personal needs but also fosters a profound sense of joy and contentment.

——— JOY PRACTICE: ———
Am I Lonely?

Loneliness is a significant health risk. Here are three questions to ask yourself right now. While the questions are based upon research at UCLA, they are not meant to be diagnostic but just to get you thinking.[3] If you are feeling lonely, reach out to a counselor or therapist who can do a proper assessment and treatment plan.

How often do you feel that you lack companionship?

- ☐ Hardly ever
- ☐ Sometimes
- ☐ Often

How often do you feel left out?

- ☐ Hardly ever
- ☐ Sometimes
- ☐ Often

How often do you feel isolated from others?

- ☐ Hardly ever
- ☐ Sometimes
- ☐ Often

While most people feel lonely at times, if you answered "often" to any of these, please take action on addressing your loneliness with a counselor or therapist.

TAKE AN INVENTORY OF YOUR CONNECTIONS

As humans, every one of us experiences the painful dance between connection and disconnection. Evolutionary psychologist Robin Dunbar explains, "Friendship and loneliness are two sides of the same social coin, and we lurch through life from one to the other." It gets even more lurchy when our friends, spouses, and relatives move or pass away.

Dr. Dunbar created an approach to fostering connections that is practical, tested, and simple: the Dunbar circle.[4] Your Dunbar circle is a bull's-eye made up of concentric circles. You are at the center of the bull's-eye. As you move out from the center, each concentric circle has more people but with less meaningful connection. The first ring out is the **close friend ring**. Here are five people that you would be comfortable calling if you had good news or bad news or needed a favor in some way. After close friends is the **good friend ring**. We see these friends less often than those in the center group, but the relationships are warm and reciprocal in some way. In the **friend ring** are typically people we've gotten to know a bit and whom we would casually call a friend but are not especially close with. Finally, the ring that consists of acquaintances is up to one hundred people that you know, but not well.

If you feel like you don't have many close friends right now, you are not alone. Having few close friends, especially later in life, is painful, but with effort, it can be temporary. No doubt you have been investing your time and effort in other important areas, like work or caregiving or just surviving. In longevity, friendships can become more of a priority.

A fascinating study of 2,013 adults, ages eighteen to seventy-five, examined three kinds of relationships (romantic, family, and friend) that impact life satisfaction. A key finding was that high-quality friendships buffer the effects of unsatisfactory intimate relationships on life satisfaction and joy. Individuals with strong friendships reported high life satisfaction even if their romantic relationships were lacking. In contrast, those satisfied with their intimate relationships experienced high life satisfaction regardless of friendship quality.

Family relationships also positively impacted life satisfaction but did not affect other relationship types as significantly, likely due to the varied nature of family ties. The takeaways are: (1) All three relationship types (romantic, friendship, and family) matter; and (2) given the fact that if you live long enough you are likely to lose your romantic partner to death or divorce, make sure to cultivate your friendships with family and friends.[5]

——— JOY PRACTICE: ———
Your Current Dunbar Circle

Draw your own current Dunbar circle and take a moment to fill it in.

- Bull's-eye: Write your name.
- Close friend ring: Jot down the names of the three to five people you are closest to.
- Good friend ring: List fifteen people who matter to you. You see them less often than those in the center group, but the relationships are warm and reciprocal in some way.
- Friend ring: This can include *up to* fifty people you know a bit and see regularly but don't count as your own friends.
- Acquaintance ring: This ring can include up to one hundred people. Jot down some names of people you know and like but are not close to.

It is okay if you struggled with your current circle. It's just a baseline from which your connections can grow.

What would be your ideal circle? Let yourself imagine what it would look like and fill in your own aspirational Dunbar circle. Go wild with it. In addition to your current connections, write those you'd like to include. You might write the name of a person (family member, friend, acquaintance, neighbor) whom you have lost contact with or someone you know and would like to know better. If you can't think of anyone, don't worry, just use a placeholder like "friend 1." You may also want to try to describe that person. For example, "someone who lives nearby that I could go to dinner with" or "someone I can call when I'm feeling down or need a ride." The very process of identifying your connection needs puts the wheels in motion for cultivating that new or renewed friendship.

IT'S NEVER TOO LATE TO MAKE FRIENDS

The idea that you are "too old" to find new friends or new love is rooted in internalized ageism. Both research and real-life stories consistently prove otherwise. Building new relationships as you go through life is normal, rewarding, and contributes to joyspan.

Adults of all ages can—and do—forge meaningful platonic and romantic relationships. Psychologist Laura Carstensen's socioemotional selectivity theory suggests that as people age, they prioritize emotionally fulfilling relationships, which may lead to more selective but deeper social bonds. Older adults are often better equipped to form meaningful connections because they are more focused on quality relationships rather than quantity.[6] So age can be an advantage in building new relationships; we have more clarity about our values, interests, and goals, which can facilitate authentic connections.

After her divorce at age sixty-eight, Andrea felt disoriented and emotionally drained. She had been married for more than thirty-five years, and her identity was deeply intertwined with her role as a wife and a mother. Suddenly, she found herself alone, questioning her worth. Andrea initially believed that her opportunity to find love or make new friends had passed, feeling "too old" and "too broken" to start again.

Despite her doubts, Andrea began attending a book club at her local library, where she met a group of women who shared her love of literature and intellectual discussions. Over time, these women became friends. They encouraged her to explore new hobbies, and together they embarked on hiking trips, cooking classes, and even a weekend getaway. These newfound friends helped Andrea rediscover her confidence and joy in life.

Encouraged by her friends, Andrea eventually tried online dating. After a few months, she met Jeff, a gentle man with a passion for the outdoors. The two connected over shared experiences and a love for adventure. Their relationship developed slowly, marked by a deep appreciation for each other's history. Andrea's relationship with Jeff showed her that love could be just as fulfilling in her later years as it was in her youth—perhaps even more so, because she had a clearer sense of who she was and what she wanted.

Age is not a barrier to emotional connection. Rebuilding your social life after loss and after heartbreak is possible. New friendships are possible. New love is possible. It is not too late and you are not too old.

HOW TO STAY CONNECTED WITH FRIENDS

Friends offer emotional support, shared history, and companionship. However, as responsibilities and life circumstances change, maintaining these relationships becomes more complex.

One of the most critical factors in maintaining friendships is consistent communication. Research underscores that regular contact is essential for sustaining relationships. Regular interactions, even brief communications, are linked to better relationship satisfaction and more lasting relationships. Friendships are maintained through "small but consistent behaviors" rather than grand gestures.[7]

Flexibility is another essential element in maintaining friendships through the years. Health changes and caregiving obligations may limit the time available for socializing. A willingness to adapt and compromise on plans is crucial. The ability to adjust expectations and accommodate each other's schedules plays a significant role in friendship longevity. For instance, you may need to try meeting for a quick coffee instead of a long lunch, or scheduling a catch-up via a phone call instead of in person. Adapting to these changes allows friendships to remain resilient.

Emotional vulnerability is also essential in maintaining friendships over the years. Psychological studies reveal that authentic friendships are built on mutual trust, understanding, and vulnerability. Friendships require emotional openness to grow deeper, which becomes particularly important as you encounter health issues, loss of a spouse, or family changes. By sharing both positive and challenging experiences, you foster trust and deepen your friendships.

Adult life is marked by transitions, which often redefine social circles and availability. Friends who understand and embrace one another's life changes tend to maintain stronger and more satisfying relationships. Support also includes commemorating life events—attending weddings, funerals, celebrating children's achievements and birthdays. By actively participating in each other's life events, friends build memories and affirm their ongoing commitment to the relationship.

Pride Aside

You know that friend who instigates connection? The one who picks up the phone just to check in? The one who is there when you need them? Be THAT friend. We often get so caught up in the fact that nobody is reaching out to us, we forget that *we* can do the reaching out. Your friends are likely to reciprocate based upon what you've modeled.

Cary hadn't expected to ever feel lonely. She'd enjoyed a long marriage, rich with travel, friends, and a satisfying career. When her husband developed dementia, he seemed to prefer napping to anything she'd suggest.

Her once-busy life slowed, and she longed for someone to talk to. After days of this quiet ache, Cary decided something had to change.

While sorting through a box of old letters one afternoon, she stumbled upon a note from her high school best friend, Kathy. The sight of Kathy's name brought back a flood of memories—late-night talks, shared secrets, and the way they'd laughed together until their sides hurt. They'd lost touch over the years, but as Cary reread Kathy's words, she felt an urge to reconnect.

Cary found Kathy's phone number online, and after taking a deep breath, she called. "Is this Kathy?" she asked in a shaky voice. Then she heard a delighted laugh, and the years melted away. They arranged to meet for coffee, and soon one meeting turned into regular lunches and dinners. Kathy introduced her to others from their old friends circle and their friendship was alive again, richer with their life stories.

Cary had spent years longing for friends to reach out, or check in, or invite her over. Now she understood that if she wanted friendships, she couldn't wait for others to make the first move.

It wasn't easy, but after reaching out to Kathy, she swallowed her pride and reached out to other friends, family members, and even acquaintances. She picked up the phone, sent handwritten notes, texts just to say hello, and invitations for coffee. Some people responded right away, others took their time, and a few didn't respond at all. But she kept reaching out.

She soon noticed a shift. Her efforts set a tone for her relationships. People began to reach out to her, following the pattern she had modeled. Her niece called her out of the blue one morning to say, "I was thinking of you." Kathy dropped by unexpectedly with a pie. The friendships she was nurturing became reciprocal, each person showing up for the other.

In the end, Cary had created the companionship she'd longed for. She found herself surrounded by people who valued her presence as much as she valued theirs. The connections she'd built felt fuller and more vibrant because she'd chosen to be "that friend" (see figure 10).

FIGURE 10. Joyspan Matrix in Action: Cary, Age 79

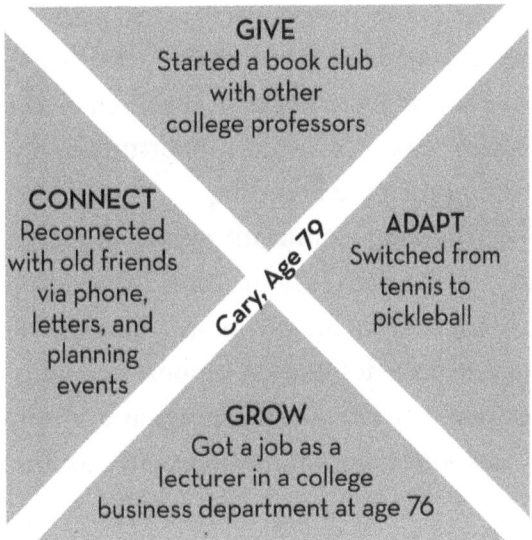

Long-Distance Friends

When friends move away or we move away from friends, friendships may wither on the vine. Fortunately, with intentional communication, planning, and a commitment to staying connected, it's possible to maintain long-distance friendships. Here are evidence-based strategies for maintaining close friendships across distances.

1. Prioritize Regular and Meaningful Communication

Research shows that regular communication is the key component of maintaining long-distance friendships. It is the quality of the communication, rather than frequency alone, that is the strongest predictor of friendship satisfaction over distance. To cultivate meaningful communication and the joy it brings, you might schedule regular "catch-up" calls where you focus solely on each other and update one another on significant life events.

2. Plan Visits and Attend Milestone Events

Spending time together in person, even occasionally, can have a lasting positive impact on friendship quality, increasing feelings of intimacy and trust. Planning visits or trips together, even if they happen only once or twice a year, provides opportunities to create shared memories that strengthen the friendship.

Additionally, attending significant events in each other's lives—such as birthday celebrations, graduations, or weddings—is helpful. Research shows that sharing life events enhances the closeness of relationships because it provides mutual support and adds depth. When distance makes frequent visits challenging, at a minimum, going to key milestone occasions is a meaningful way to sustain the friendship over time.

3. Cultivate Shared Experiences Through Technology

Technology offers creative ways to bridge the long-distance friendship gap. Video chats, online gaming, and streaming services allow you to engage in activities simultaneously, even if you're miles apart. For example, "watch parties" enable you to watch shows together and chat in real time, re-creating the experience of watching together in the same room. Friends who enjoy gaming can play online, multiplayer games, fostering teamwork and friendly competition. Additionally, reading the same book, cooking a recipe together via a video call, or joining a virtual class can create new shared memories and help maintain a strong connection.

4. Practice Active Listening and Emotional Support

Providing emotional support and practicing active listening are essential components of close friendships. In long-distance relationships, the lack of face-to-face interaction can make these skills even more crucial.

When you are physically apart, misunderstandings are more likely, so being attentive and empathetic during conversations is essential.

To maintain emotional closeness, prioritize listening and show genuine interest in each other's lives. Ask open-ended questions, express empathy, and validate each other's feelings to build trust and show that you care, even from afar. The "emotional bank account" theory suggests that small acts of kindness, such as offering encouragement or remembering important dates, contribute to emotional intimacy over time.[8] Like a financial bank account, relationships thrive on deposits and withdrawals. Deposits are positive actions—such as kindness, honesty, and dependability—that build trust and goodwill, while withdrawals—such as disrespect or broken promises—diminish trust. Thinking of friendship in terms of an emotional bank account highlights the importance of small, consistent positive actions to sustain your relationships.

5. Maintain a Positive Mindset and Avoid Resentment

Long-distance friendships are more successful when you both approach the relationship with a positive mindset. A common challenge in long-distance friendships is the feeling of resentment when one person perceives that the other isn't putting in enough effort. Communication about expectations and feelings is key to avoiding this type of resentment.

It's helpful to acknowledge that there will be times when life gets busy and communication may slow down. By discussing this possibility openly, you can prevent misunderstandings and encourage each other to reach out without guilt. Approaching the friendship with a sense of understanding and patience allows both people to feel secure and valued, even when distance creates logistical challenges.

Regular and meaningful communication, low-pressure exchanges, planned visits, shared virtual experiences, active listening, and a positive mindset are all strategies that help friends stay close despite physical separation.

HOW TO FIND NEW FRIENDS

Paige had been married to Andy for fifty-one years. "After Andy died, my social life was…crickets," sighed Paige. "I felt it most on the weekend nights especially. I didn't want to be a third wheel with our couple friends, and I didn't want to hang any guilt on my adult children. I thought maybe I'd just be lonely forever."

Fortunately, Paige decided to try to make new friends. The first week she went to farmers markets, talked to a few people, and scored some fantastic pomegranate juice. The second week she went to an antique car show, which was interesting but attended by mostly men. The third week she went to the nearby dog park. "I didn't have a dog, but I do like them," she confided and laughed. "I sat down at a bench so the big ones wouldn't knock me over." At first, she just sat and watched people mingle while their dogs played. It wasn't too long before the dogs romped her way and their owners followed. As dogs approached, she commented on the kind eyes of the golden retriever, the head tilt of the Jack Russell terrier, the poof of the black poodle. The owners would then tell her about how Ollie loved strangers, or Hudson was a rescue, or Lucky was nearly blind.

A few days later, Paige visited the same dog park and, recognizing her, a pet owner, Courtney, guided her dog right over to her shady bench. This time, in addition to dog talk, they also talked about other things and exchanged names and a few laughs. After a couple of additional chats, Paige invited Courtney for a coffee. Newly divorced, Courtney was delighted. Ten years later the two are good friends and, in fact, Courtney was the maid of honor for Paige's wedding. Paige had met her new husband at an animal rescue event.

Potential new connections, both platonic and romantic, are all around you once you start looking. Invite a neighbor over to watch the *Academy Awards*. Bring doughnuts to a volunteer event. Join a knitting circle, a salsa class, or maybe a writing workshop. If you pursue your interests, friends will follow, and they will likely be kindred spirits.

> "You might have to kiss a lot of frogs before you find your people. But keep going, you'll find them. Don't wait. These future friends are lonely too. They need you to make the first move."
>
> —*Betty, age ninety-six*

Micro Connections

One of the best ways to make new friends is to make micro connections throughout the day. Everywhere you go—a coffee shop, the supermarket, et cetera—try to connect with others. Smile at someone, say hello, or pay them an authentic compliment. Micro connections work a connection muscle in us, and they can grow into bigger connections.

As my older neighbor Marina likes to say, "A smile opens the door. A friendly greeting is an entry to friendship." She makes micro connections with her favorite team members at Whole Foods, the staff at medical appointments, and people at the hairdresser. Sometimes relationships are built on long, meaningful conversations, but other times, they are based upon a brief shared laugh.

Rekindling

When we were younger, friendships occurred by default. In grade school, we'd sit next to someone with the same bag of chips. You have that kind of chips? I have that kind of chips! Friendship made. Who was your closest pal from elementary school? Your mischievous high school friends? Your hip college friends? Your uniform-wearing friends from work? The friends you made pacing the sidelines of the football field? If you don't know now how they all are, where they are, or even what their names were, you are normal. I've yet to meet a human who has successfully maintained every friendship they've ever made. We're all in the same *drifted friendships* boat.

If you feel fewer social connections as you grow older, these drifters might be a good place to start expanding your friend circle. It takes far less detective work these days to find someone you've lost touch with. I typed my best elementary friend's maiden name into Facebook, and she popped right up. You can also try Instagram, LinkedIn, or TikTok. I sent this Facebook message to my friend: "Hi, Jill! It's Kerry Parker. I came across your profile today, and it brought a big smile to my face. How can it have been forty years? I'd love to catch up and hope all is well. With love, Kerry." She responded, and then we caught up on the phone. We live in different states now, but she told me about a mutual friend who still lives in California, and I reached out to her as well. Two more friends were added to my social portfolio: one via phone; one in person. Imagine doing this with all your drifters!

Diversify Your Social Portfolio

A key principle of investing is to diversify your financial portfolio: Don't invest all your money in the same thing. This principle is equally true for our social portfolios: Don't put all your friends in the same basket. In the second half of life, we lose friends to the big Ds: distance, disease, dementia, and death. This results in another D—it's disheartening. If you diversify your friendships by having friends of different ages and at different stages, you increase your odds of a full and lasting social life. But how?

Here's how seventy-one-year-old Margo diversified her social portfolio. "I was a leader at work and had a ton of friends. I retired three years ago, and I've already lost touch with almost everyone," Margo explained. "My other friends are spread about the country, and since my divorce five years ago, it feels harder to hang out with my 'couple' friends as well."

Realizing that her social network was taking a nosedive, Margo decided to approach her friendship situation as if it were a work project. First, she wrote out a list of things she was interested in: photography, gardening, hiking, and reading. For each interest, she wrote down three ideas. For example, under photography she wrote: "Photography 101 class at Saddleback Community College"; "photographers group on the online Meetup site"; and the "Festival of the Arts photography exhibits." She did this with each interest, and then took a highlighter to flag what she'd tackle first. She started with the online Meetup group. It was all these people who were interested in photography who met in person each week at various locations. "What a dynamic heterogeneous group, and we had so much to share in terms of our learning and frustrations with photography." Margo especially clicked with a person who'd attended her college alma mater. They laughed that they'd missed each other in college (by twenty-seven years) but picked right up as if they'd been classmates.

FAMILY CONNECTIONS IN OLDER AGE

Typically defined by blood ties or legal connections (siblings, in-laws, adult children, grandchildren, extended family), family relationships can be an especially important component of your social portfolio as you grow older. Unlike friendships, which are chosen and may come and go, family connections are typically enduring and can provide a safety net in the hard times. Family relationships can involve deep-seated emotional bonds but often carry unresolved tensions and expectations. Something I've quickly learned as a gerontologist is that there are no perfect families, and all family relationships take work, forgiveness, and compromise.

Creating, maintaining, and repairing family bonds all are vital to joyspan and take work. This section delves into the essential components of building family connection: authentic interest; shared fun; open communication; family routines; and openness to technology. Family connections are more than a source of comfort; they can impact the quality of your longevity by bolstering resilience and meaning.

Authentic Interest

One of the most effective ways to cultivate and sustain family connections is to demonstrate a deep and genuine interest in your family members' lives. When you express curiosity, your family members feel valued and understood. Studies indicate that people who feel genuinely listened to and appreciated by family members are more likely to maintain strong, positive relationships.[9] When you actively engage with family members, inquire about their lives, and listen empathetically, you strengthen your role within the family. This interest may be expressed in small gestures, like asking about work or hobbies, or in more profound conversations, such as sharing life experiences and personal challenges. These interactions enhance trust, emotional closeness, and satisfaction within family relationships. Get creative in which family members you reach out to: your sister, sure, but how about your sister's child or grandchild?

Genuine interest is also linked to empathy, an essential component of healthy family relationships. Empathy has been shown to lower stress levels in both the giver and the receiver, promoting emotional resilience and reducing family conflicts. For older adults, this empathy-based approach to connection can transform family interactions into enriching, supportive experiences that contribute to better mental health and life satisfaction.

For older adults, maintaining an authentic interest in family members also enhances their sense of generativity, or the desire to contribute positively to the lives of younger generations. When you show interest in your loved ones, you actively participate in the growth and well-being of the family unit. Studies show that older adults who invest energy in building connections with younger family members have lower rates of depression, better cognitive functioning, and increased feelings of self-worth.

Make It Fun

When thinking about phone calls, letters, video calls, or visits with family members of different ages, fun matters. Here are some ideas and tips on how to make family interactions memorable and fun for all:

- **Try hands-on activities.** In person or on a video call, try doing something you like... together. You may want to bake cookies, paint, carve, or play the same instrument with a grandchild or other family member.
- **Incorporate storytelling.** Sharing tales from your childhood, family anecdotes, or stories about when parents were young is a memorable way to connect. My friend Cary stashes old photos in her pocket and whips them out at family parties and has everyone in stitches with the story she tells about a particular photo.
- **Plan a mini-adventure or an outing.** It can be a simple walk to the park or a nearby coffee shop. If staying in is more practical, you can create adventures at home by setting up a treasure hunt, camping in the backyard, or transforming your living

room into a movie theater complete with popcorn and cozy blankets.

Making your time together special doesn't have to be elaborate; sometimes it's the little things that leave the biggest impression. Create simple traditions with family members like a special breakfast you cook together or a game only you play. For young family members, these rituals create a sense of excitement and familiarity. Embracing these moments will not only make visits enjoyable but will also strengthen the special bond that only family can offer.

Open Up

Communication is key to maintaining strong family relationships, especially as family dynamics evolve over time. Open communication is a form of dialogue where all parties feel safe, respected, and encouraged to express their thoughts, feelings, and concerns honestly and without fear of judgment. It emphasizes listening actively, showing empathy, and fostering mutual understanding. Studies highlight that open communication can help families navigate health issues, changing living arrangements, and financial concerns. Open communication also reduces misunderstandings that can lead to family conflict. Families with open communication report higher levels of satisfaction and cohesion, as each member feels heard and valued.[10]

I had the benefit of a beautiful example of open communication between Betty and one of her fifteen grandchildren. Her grandson called, and because we were driving, I got to hear both sides of the conversation on the speakerphone.

The grandson said, "Momo, no matter how hard I work in school, I can't keep up." Betty responded, "I'm so sorry you're feeling that way, sweetie. Can you tell me more about what's been hardest for you?" He sighed before continuing, "It's everything—classes, exams, and balancing it all with my part-time job. I'm constantly behind and I hate it so bad."

Betty replied, "That sounds really tough. I'm so proud of you for juggling so much. Is there anything I can do to help? Even if it's just being here to listen or helping you brainstorm solutions?" He told her about some things he was trying and then said, "Honestly, just talking to you helps." Betty smiled, saying, "I'm glad I can help, and we can figure this out together—I'm always here for you."

The grandmother showed empathy, and the grandson felt safe. The conversation was collaborative, with no blame or criticism, which is key, as no one likes to be judged, and no one is in the mood for a lecture.

Family Routines

Maintaining consistent family routines or traditions is another great way to strengthen bonds. Regular interactions, such as weekly phone calls, family dinners, or shared, scheduled activities, help reinforce family cohesion. Setting up regular times for these things helps create a reliable pattern of communication. Your rituals can be as simple as a Sunday phone call or as elaborate as a yearly family reunion. Creating family routines encourages shared experiences, which are integral to bonding. Even virtual activities, like watching a movie together online or having a family game night via video call, can foster closeness. If your family does not yet have a dedicated time in place, why not be the one to initiate it?

Embrace Technology

These days, staying close to family members doesn't have to require any travel. You can get quite creative by using technology for quality connection.

Although the various and ever-changing communication options often require a learning curve, you can do it. If you have trouble getting set up, ask friends and relatives for help, check whether your local library offers tutorials, and find online instruction via Google or YouTube videos.

Adults who learn to use digital communication tools experience reduced feelings of isolation and improved mental health. Video calls, social media, and messaging apps enable us to maintain frequent contact with family members, fostering a sense of closeness despite physical distance.

That's how Lisa, who ran a booming pet food business in Arizona, benefited from technology. Lisa retired and was eager to reconnect with friends from high school and college, work friends, and, most of all, her two nieces and a nephew.

Her youngest niece, now twenty-seven, lives in Oregon; while her other niece, twenty-nine, lives in California. Her nephew, thirty-five, lives in Scotland with his wife and three-year-old son. Lisa reached out to each one and asked, "What's your favorite way to keep in touch? Text messaging, FaceTime, in person, et cetera?"

Her Oregon niece preferred in-person visits. The niece in California favored texting because it kept her connected to everyone, all the time. Her nephew said he loved FaceTime and WhatsApp. Lisa made a note of their preferences. She resisted the urge to ask, "What's WhatsApp?" Instead, she searched online for WhatsApp and easily followed the instructions. She was able to message her nephew in Scotland for free, asking about his wife and their baby and for him to send photos. When she learned that he loved dogs, she sent a photo of her golden retriever and then mailed a golden retriever stuffed animal for the baby. After that, she called her niece in Oregon to pick a time and place to visit in person. In the meantime, she texted the California niece to ask about graduate school and surf lessons. These family members are delighted to reconnect with their "cool aunt Lisa," and their mother was touched that Lisa was getting to know her kids as adults. Win-win.

Now that we've explored the first joytank, growth, and the second joytank, connection, the next chapter explores the third joytank, adapting to life's shifts as we age.

JOYSPANNER: Jimmy Carter

Former US President Jimmy Carter, born in 1924, was known for his humility, integrity, faith, and strong relationships with family, friends, colleagues, and those he served. Mr. Carter was the first president to reach one hundred years of age before he passed away in 2024. He attributed his longevity to his faith, a strong sense of purpose, staying mentally active, and strong family relationships.

> **GROW:** Early in life, Carter was a peanut farmer. In middle age he served as president, and as an older man he was a global humanitarian. His willingness to adapt and take on new roles allowed him to impact countless lives, demonstrating that growth and purpose can be lifelong endeavors.
>
> **CONNECT:** Carter's life was deeply enriched by his relationships with others. His enduring marriage to Rosalynn Carter, which spanned more than seventy-seven years, is a testament to the strength of his personal connections. Carter remained close with his four children and their spouses, as well as his twenty-two grandchildren and great-grandchildren. He had friends of all ages with whom he remained close before he passed.

ADAPT: Carter adapted to the changing needs of the world, shifting his focus from politics to humanitarian work and peace building. His adaptability steered him to become a global advocate for peace and human rights, mediating conflicts, monitoring elections, and addressing public health crises. Even in his nineties, Carter embraced change, continuing his work with the Carter Center and advocating for issues that impact people globally.

GIVE: Through the Carter Center, he worked to eradicate diseases, promote peace, and protect human rights, impacting millions of lives. He was also a committed volunteer for Habitat for Humanity, with whom he helped build and renovate homes, often working alongside the families who would live in them. His life was driven by his compassion and a deep sense of responsibility to help others.

President Carter's life exemplifies how dedication to service, close relationships, and a willingness to grow and adapt can create a long joyspan.

CHAPTER 6

Adapt with Joy

Howie and Beth Martin had dinner at their son's house every Wednesday night. Their son, Ira, his wife, and their two children lived forty minutes away from the senior Martins. The couple drove to the weekly dinners full of anticipation and drove home afterward chuckling at the antics of the grandchildren. In their mid-eighties, diminished eyesight made the nighttime drive too dicey to continue. With Wednesday dinners in jeopardy, the couple debated their options: give up the cherished tradition or find a way to make it work. Beth researched drivers (too expensive); Ubers (not available in their rural locations); buses (timing was off); and at last, trains. Beth studied the schedules and was delighted to find a round trip that would work. Ira could pick his parents up at the train station while his wife put the finishing touches on dinner.

One Wednesday, a heavy snowstorm delayed Ira on his way to the train. The Martins stood stranded on the platform in whipping wind and snow. Howie called his son...no answer. As his fingers grew freezing cold, he dialed his daughter-in-law...again no answer. As the couple huddled together for warmth, Beth noticed a pizza parlor across the street. Carefully, the octogenarians made their way through the storm to the restaurant. They ordered a pizza to be delivered to their son's address. Then, in a stroke of adaptive genius, Beth asked, "When you deliver it, may we ride along in the car?"

With a big smile, the delivery driver agreed, and the Martins climbed into the cozy back seat along with the steaming pizza. Laughing at the unexpected adventure, they made it to Wednesday night dinner safely, and with dinner in tow. Decades later, the Martin grandchildren still laugh as they recount this testament to their grandparents' adaptability.

> "There is nothing wrong with life itself. It is the ocean in which we swim and we either adapt to it or sink to the bottom. But it is in our power as human beings not to pollute the waters of life, not to destroy the spirit which animates us."
> —Henry Miller, writer

The third element in the Joyspan Matrix is to adapt: to adjust to a new circumstance, condition, or environment in a way that ensures continued functionality. Adaptation requires flexibility, creativity, and the ability to learn from and respond to change.

For example, maybe you love to garden but both knees now scream when you squat down. You can choose to retract by giving up gardening OR you can adapt by gardening in raised planters or posts. Let's say you love dancing, but your dance partner died. To adapt, you'd sign up for a dance class at the community center; to retract, you'd hang up your dancing shoes. The examples are endless, because growing older inevitably brings new events and conditions. You will experience retirement, changes in health, the loss of loved ones, and evolving social roles. Choosing to adapt enables you to face transitions with resilience, finding new ways to participate in life. You don't deny the challenges of getting older, but you embrace the opportunities for growth, reinvention, and joy that aging offers.

CHANGING CIRCUMSTANCES

As you age, you will encounter shifts in every direction: relationships, roles, health, transportation options, and living arrangements. You can't foresee what lies ahead, but one thing is certain: Knowing how to adapt is a key to enjoying your long life. Your response to change will determine your ability to thrive. Consider the most common circumstances that occur in later years:

Becoming a grandparent. Worldwide, there are over 1.5 billion grandparents, making this transition one of the most common experiences of later life. In the UK there are an estimated 14 million grandparents and 75 per cent of adults will likely become grandparents.[1] As families evolve, the ability to embrace shifting roles—whether as a mentor or as a babysitter—highlights the importance of adaptability in creating and maintaining intergenerational bonds.

Changes in work life. One in five retirees have difficulty adjusting to their retirement.[2] The challenges include reduced income, altered social roles, and boredom. Difficulty adjusting to retirement is not unusual. A study in Japan showed that 60 percent of wives of Japanese retirees were suffering depression, anxiety, and malaise, a condition researchers dubbed "retired husband syndrome."[3] The ability to adapt to a new work status is the difference between enjoying or lamenting this phase of life.

Uncoupling. According to the Office for National Statistics, the likelihood of living alone increases as we get older.[4] When you live a very long life, the odds are that you'll outlive your partner and your friends. This reality, plus uncoupling via divorce and separation, highlights the incredible importance of our ability to adapt to huge life changes. This requires either forming new partnerships or embracing singlehood.

Medical diagnoses. Health problems play a role in nearly every long life. A diagnosis (for you, your partner, your friends, your kids, or your grandkids) can reshape or completely transform daily routines. Learning to continue to make the most of your time while adjusting to a chronic or acute condition requires you to adapt with intention, flexibility, and grit.

Moving. Whether downsizing or relocating to be closer to family, moving involves far more than packing boxes. It requires the ability to leave behind the familiarity of a home and community, and the proactive decision to find a way to adapt to a new adventure.

Caregiving. More than one hundred million people all over the world are providing care to someone. Odds are, you will join the ranks during some portion of your life. Taking on the role of a caregiver requires tremendous adaptability to balance emotional, physical, and financial responsibilities.

Dependence. In longevity, changes in mobility due to injury or illness lead to a reliance on family, friends, or paid assistance. These changes are challenging because you have to adjust to being a recipient rather than a giver. This dilemma of dependency will require you to find new ways to maintain agency and dignity. Adaptation is indispensable to navigating dependence, to focus on what remains rather than on what is lost.

If considering facing common circumstances in later life feels daunting, that's the point. Maximizing joyspan means that you confront the inevitability of change and fortify yourself internally for the journey. Successfully adapting to change is a choice and a skill that will enable you to find new paths forward.

HOW YOU ADAPT

My friend Liz was the rock of her family. She made the travel plans, hosted the holiday meals, and grew vegetables, all while running a successful consulting practice. Last December on her way out to get the newspaper, she slipped on the icy sidewalk. Her fractured hip required surgery, months of rehabilitation, and a wheelchair.

Liz felt frustrated, defeated, and ashamed. She needed help getting out of bed, getting into bed, and everything in between. She hated asking for assistance and felt like a burden. While grieving the loss of her old way of life, Liz reluctantly allowed herself to accept help. A neighbor brought her groceries once a week, her granddaughter set up a home office for Liz from her bed, and an aide and physiotherapist came regularly.

With time, Liz realized that her dependence didn't erase her value. The new circumstance meant she needed to adapt. She turned her attention to what remained—her love of her family, her sharp mind, and her determined spirit. Her family and friends weren't just helping her; they were collaborating with her as she created a new chapter of life.

My mother, Betty, is a master adapter. Well-meaning acquaintances and neighbors have advised her "to move out of that treacherous two-story house. You are ninety-six, after all!" One of her neighbors went so far as to ask me how I will feel when she falls down the stairs. But Betty says, "Everyone is different in what is best for them when they grow old. For me, because I've been lucky enough to live with my mind intact, living at home is what I want. It brings me joy every single day. In my case, living here at home is well worth the risk of falling. It is my choice."

While living alone in your nineties is neither possible nor desirable for many people, it was very much the right choice for Betty. She navigates her external environment like a rock star. She puts in the thought and the effort to adapt to the everyday hurdles of growing older. For example, with scoliosis, double knee replacements, a hip replacement, and severe osteoarthritis, Betty's mobility is very limited and painful. Yet she doesn't have a bedroom downstairs; she loves to prepare her meals, but supermarkets require a ton of walking; and her home is filled with hard, unforgiving floors, stairs, and sharp edges.

Here's how she has adapted to each of these circumstances. No bedroom downstairs? "I have a pretty nifty couch downstairs that I can sleep on, and I've saved up for this new kind of less-expensive lift," she explains. Her pain level is too great for her to walk for exercise, so Betty has adapted by using a stationary bike at the lowest level each day. In addition to the pedaling, she knows that weight training is a must, but she didn't have weights and didn't know which exercises were safe to do. She asked her doctor about physiotherapy, and he agreed it was a good idea. She attends two sessions of physiotherapy every week and repeats the moves at home each day. After she turned ninety-five, her driving was curtailed and getting to physiotherapy became a problem. Her adaptation trick? Finding a physiotherapy company covered by insurance that would come to her home.

Getting to the supermarket also became a problem, partially because of driving but mostly because of the size of the supermarkets in her area. "It felt like walking the length of a football field just to go get some milk," Betty laments. She solved that obstacle by ordering groceries online for home delivery. This was not a one-and-done endeavor, however. It took many sessions to navigate the very unfamiliar world of online shopping, and the process was peppered with trials and errors. Still, more and more innovative solutions exist for those willing to grapple with new technology that is outside their comfort zones.

What about getting around in a house filled with fall hazards and hard floors? Betty always had her hand on a wall to steady herself.

When this was no longer enough to feel secure, she had to confront her resistance to using a walker. She couldn't see herself hunched over an ugly walker with tennis balls on it. Happily, walkers have evolved with modern designs that are both useful and even cool (they come in red, too!). Betty found a triangular model that is lightweight and has a pocket for carrying items from place to place. At first, she used the walker only at home, but soon she grew so comfortable with it that she ventured outside. In the years to come, Betty may require a wheelchair, but I have no doubt that she'll navigate the transition with equal grit and coping skills.

Here's an example of how Betty adapted to an emotional burden. She was in her seventies when her son, Russ, was diagnosed with acute myelogenous leukemia. She couldn't sleep and couldn't stop shaking. The feelings were sharp, frantic, and accompanied by debilitating anxiety. Everyday tasks felt impossible to complete because her mind was foggy, and her thoughts were racing. It felt out of sequence to be in good health while her son was fighting for his life.

Betty allowed herself to feel it all and put in the daily and at times daunting work of adapting to this new very abnormal normal. Betty allowed her wisest daughter, my sister KC, and me to serve as supports for her in her great anguish. In turn, Betty became a support for her daughter-in-law, Karen, whom she loves just like a daughter. Karen was caring for their three young children while navigating the seemingly endless challenges of Russ's chemotherapy, radiation, and a bone marrow transplant. During this time, it was important for Karen, Russ, their children, Betty, and all the rest of us to feel and express our big emotions. Studies consistently show that people who suppress or ignore their feelings often experience worse psychological outcomes than those who recognize and express their emotions.[5] Feelings don't follow a linear trajectory. Renowned psychiatrist Elisabeth Kübler-Ross originally identified five stages of grief—denial, anger, bargaining, depression, and acceptance—but even she clarified later in her career that these stages were not linear or universally applicable. Instead, feelings occur and recur unpredictably. Adapting to change in circumstances is less about moving on and more about adjusting to a new way of experiencing life.

Many years have passed since Russ's leukemia diagnosis. The hospital where Russ received his treatment hosts a big outdoor picnic event every year. Patients and former patients who have had bone marrow transplantations attend the picnic along with their friends and family members. Attendees who have undergone the bone marrow transplant wear a large circular pin with the number of years it has been since they received the lifesaving transplant. My brother's pin reads "15." Our mother attends the picnics and though there is no pin for her ability to adapt to the life-threatening illness of her son, that is certainly pin-worthy. Your ability to adapt is pin-worthy, too!

HOW TO HELP SOMEONE DURING A LIFE CHANGE

Supporting someone going through a challenging time isn't easy. Being there (physically or through other means of communication) makes all the difference, even if you're unsure of what to say. Your compassion and understanding are more valuable than finding any "right" words.

Listen: Avoid changing the subject or minimizing the loss. Instead, acknowledge the situation and allow the person to talk and vent, free of judgment. Listening is more important than speaking.

Give practical assistance: Instead of vague offers of help, suggest specific tasks you can take on, like grocery shopping, cooking, or household chores. People may not feel motivated to ask for help in rough times, so make your assistance concrete and tangible.

Keep up the support: Continue to check in periodically. When someone is going through a troubling diagnosis, a loss, or a new part of life, there isn't a known end date to the associated challenges, just changes in how they are feeling.

Watch for warning signs of depression: If a loved one's grief or fear worsens or doesn't gradually improve, this may indicate depression or anxiety. Be supportive and, if necessary, encourage them to seek professional help.

JOY PRACTICE:
Feeling the Feelings

When you are drowning in the quicksand of relentless change, grief, or loss, everything feels overwhelming and paralyzing. Here are a few ideas to implement when you don't know what to do.

REFLECT AND WRITE

- Jot down a few sentences about the grief you are feeling or a memory of your loved one.
- Optional: Write a short "letter" to your lost loved one sharing a thought or moment from your day.

BREATHE AND GROUND

- Take five slow breaths, inhaling deeply for a count of four and exhaling for a count of four.
- Place your hand over your heart or close your eyes to feel more grounded.

Fresh Air Break

- Step outside for fresh air or a short walk, noticing one or two things around you—a tree, the sky, a flower. Then close your eyes and notice a few things you can hear or smell.

Text a Supportive Friend

- Text or call someone who is a good listener. Let them know you're thinking about your loved one or need a quick chat.
- These brief, manageable exercises can help you cope with just about anything in a gentle and practical way, providing moments of calm and connection throughout your day. Use any or all of them as often as you need.

HOW TO COPE

Harry graduated from Stanford and served as a Green Beret. His story, like yours and mine, is a tapestry of highs and lows. What set Harry apart was his remarkable ability to adapt after life knocked him to the ground. Not only did Harry allow me to share his story—he insisted I share it. He hoped that through his experiences, you might find inspiration to adapt to life's challenges.

When Harry was seven years old, he heard planes roaring over his home in Hawaii on their way to bomb Pearl Harbor. The day he turned eighteen, Harry joined the military. With the help of the G.I. Bill, he attended college, where he met and married Joan. The couple had one daughter, Rose.

At twenty-one, Rose had a falling-out with her mother and became estranged from both parents. She didn't see them throughout Joan's battle with Alzheimer's disease, nor did she attend Joan's funeral. After Joan's death, Harry was deeply lonely.

Harry was also vulnerable. He began to receive daily phone calls from "new friends" and "charity organizations." Sixteen months later, Harry had given away $400,000 and his home was in foreclosure. He'd been scammed out of his life savings. Despondent over the situation, Harry ended up in the hospital. He was admitted for malnourishment and dehydration, but the deeper cause was financial exploitation.

I met Harry at the hospital while working at the Elder Abuse Forensic Center. During our interview, Harry explained, "After Joan died, I was a boat without a rudder. For the first time in my life, I was a mark. These shady characters saw an opportunity and pounced on me." Happily, that is not the end of Harry's story.

Here's how Harry got his groove back—and how you can, too. Harry employed coping strategies to manage the internal and external demands of his situation.

Internal Strategies

Harry adapted by using a combination of internal and external strategies. Internal coping strategies come from within and are the mental and emotional approaches you use to handle adversity. For example, Harry used journaling and meditation to process his emotions and try to make sense of the series of events that he'd gone through. He also used cognitive restructuring to reframe how he looked at the situation. Harry was experiencing tremendous shame over losing his home and life savings to the scam artists who reached him through the telephone. With time and effort, Harry adjusted his thinking to place the shame on the criminals who prey on people when they are most vulnerable.

Practices such as self-kindness and gratitude cultivate positivity, reinforcing emotional resilience. Relaxation techniques like deep breathing calm your nervous system, and creative hobbies provide an outlet for expression and a sense of accomplishment.

Setting small, achievable goals and maintaining routines can help establish stability and a sense of progress during times of uncertainty. Pouring yourself into the ordinary can be priceless. Summarized below are some useful tools to help you adapt to stress, loss, and change.

Internal Coping Strategies

Internal Coping Strategy	How It Helps	What Psychologists Call This
Journal to process your emotions.	Helps you recognize, understand, and manage emotions effectively.	Emotional regulation
Practice self-kindness.	Encourages treating yourself with the same compassion you would show to a friend.	Self-compassion
Meditate.	Reduces stress, increases mindfulness, and enhances emotional resilience.	Mindfulness practice
Gratitude practice.	Encourages a positive outlook by recognizing what's going well in life.	Positive reappraisal
Deep breathing exercises.	Helps calm the nervous system and reduce feelings of anxiety.	Relaxation techniques
Create something.	Provides an outlet for emotional expression and fosters a sense of accomplishment.	Expressive therapy
Set small, achievable goals.	Boosts confidence and motivation by fostering a sense of progress.	Goal-setting

Reframe the problem.	Challenges negative thought patterns and replaces them with more hopeful perspectives.	Cognitive restructuring
Keep a routine.	Establishes a sense of normalcy and stability during times of change.	Behavioral activation
Practice visualization.	Imagining positive outcomes helps reduce stress and build optimism.	Imagery rescripting

External Strategies

It is hard, if not impossible, to carry the weight of change and loss alone. External coping strategies tap into resources beyond yourself. In Harry's loneliness as a widower, he needed the support of friends and family. Without that support, Harry was vulnerable to exploitation.

Having lost his house, Harry moved into a board and care home with five other older adults. Harry was the only resident without cognitive impairment. "My roommates were nice enough, but I needed to get out of there during the day," he told me. He found a volunteer position at an equestrian therapy center for special-needs children, where his job was to meet the kids when they arrived. Harry greeted them and offered them a snack while they waited for their time to ride. Volunteering is not only great for continued growth, but it can also be helpful in adapting to loss or other changes in later life.

Spiritual and religious gatherings also often provide comfort through shared practices and beliefs, and Harry started attending church regularly. Another external coping strategy he employed was seeking professional support. Regular counseling sessions gave Harry tailored guidance for managing not only his grief as a widower, but also the stress that resulted from the financial exploitation and the trauma from losing his home. Here is a list of external coping strategies.

External Coping Strategies

External Coping Strategy	How It Helps	What Psychologists Call It
Seek support from friends and family.	Provides emotional validation and practical help during challenging times.	Social support
Join a support group.	Creates a sense of community and reduces feelings of isolation.	Peer support
Volunteer for a cause.	Enhances purpose and connects you with others while benefiting the community.	Altruistic engagement
Consult a therapist or a counselor.	Offers professional guidance for managing stress and emotions.	Psychotherapy
Attend religious or spiritual gatherings.	Builds a sense of purpose and belonging through shared practices.	Spiritual community support
Take a class or learn a new skill.	Provides a sense of accomplishment and promotes cognitive engagement.	Lifelong learning
Engage in physical activity with others.	Combines social interaction with the benefits of exercise.	Group-based exercise
Participate in community events.	Reduces isolation by building connections with neighbors and peers.	Community engagement

| Rely on trusted advisers for decision-making. | Helps manage stress by delegating responsibilities and gaining clarity. | Practical support |
| Use online forums or social media groups. | Provides access to shared experiences and advice from others facing similar challenges. | Virtual social support |

When he was devastated by life's circumstances, Harry's internal and external coping strategies fostered psychological resilience. He learned to adapt, and in doing so, he extended his joyspan. Harry's eventual celebration of life was delightfully packed with children from the riding center, and with people like me who learned from him. I had a front-row seat to the power of adapting to life's challenges (see figure 11).

FIGURE 11. Joyspan Matrix in Action: Harry, Age 82

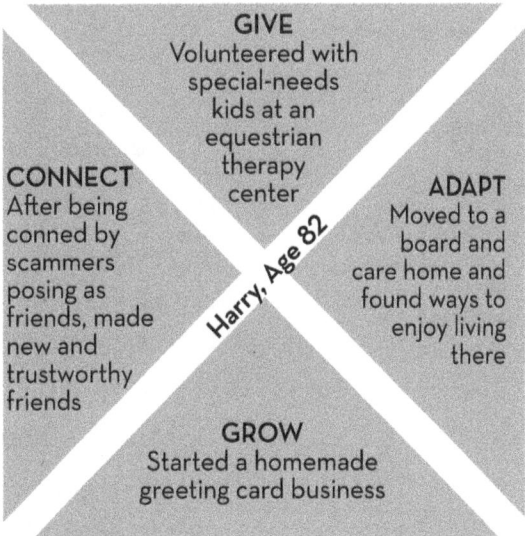

144 WHAT STRENGTHENS YOUR JOYSPAN

——— JOY PRACTICE: ———
Your Coping Strategies Toolbox

Your coping strategies toolbox contains ideas for internal and external actions to take when you are coping with a very hard time or a difficult transition. Check whether you have tried that strategy and whether it was helpful.

Internal Coping Strategy	*Tried It*
Journal to process your emotions.	☐ Yes ☐ No If so, was it helpful?
Practice self-kindness.	☐ Yes ☐ No If so, was it helpful?
Meditate.	☐ Yes ☐ No If so, was it helpful?
Gratitude practice.	☐ Yes ☐ No ☐ If so, was it helpful?
Deep breathing exercises.	☐ Yes ☐ No ☐ If so, was it helpful?
Create something.	☐ Yes ☐ No ☐ If so, was it helpful?
Set small, achievable goals.	☐ Yes ☐ No ☐ If so, was it helpful?
Reframe the problem.	☐ Yes ☐ No ☐ If so, was it helpful?
Keep a routine.	☐ Yes ☐ No ☐ If so, was it helpful?
Practice visualization.	☐ Yes ☐ No ☐ If so, was it helpful?

External Coping Strategy	Tried It
Seek support from friends and family.	☐ Yes ☐ No ☐ If so, was it helpful?
Join a support group.	☐ Yes ☐ No ☐ If so, was it helpful?
Volunteer for a cause.	☐ Yes ☐ No ☐ If so, was it helpful?
Consult a therapist or a counselor.	☐ Yes ☐ No ☐ If so, was it helpful?
Religious or spiritual gatherings.	☐ Yes ☐ No ☐ If so, was it helpful?
Take a class or learn a new skill.	☐ Yes ☐ No ☐ If so, was it helpful?
Work out with others.	☐ Yes ☐ No ☐ If so, was it helpful?
Community events.	☐ Yes ☐ No ☐ If so, was it helpful?
Trusted advisers for decision-making.	☐ Yes ☐ No ☐ If so, was it helpful?
Online community groups.	☐ Yes ☐ No ☐ If so, was it helpful?

HOW TO BOUNCE BACK

Resilience is the ability to bounce back from adversity. Witnessing resilience in people like Harry is one of the most rewarding parts of being a gerontologist. Jen is another example.

Jen's husband, Tim, died suddenly of a heart attack when they were both seventy-two years old. I'll never forget how she looked the day I met her. She sat on her couch staring at the television—except the television wasn't on. Seven months after Tim's death, Jen was diagnosed with early-stage breast cancer.

During this time, she started to write. With raw honesty, she'd write in a notebook or in letters to Tim, pouring her feelings of abandonment and fear onto the pages. Over time, the letters and journal entries evolved into reflections of gratitude—memories of their life together and the blessings she still had. Writing helped Jen understand her emotions and allowed her to grieve deeply but purposefully.

In addition to writing, she started a daily meditation and stretching practice. It was hard at first, but she stayed with it and developed a mantra that she repeated many times as she settled into the stillness: "I am strong. I am here. I am enough." The practice gave her a sense of calm and control amid the turbulence.

Social support also played a vital role in Jen's resilience. She had to push herself a bit to reach out to her sons, all of whom lived in different states. She didn't want to be "a burden" on them. Although they couldn't be with her in person, they were a good source of support and encouragement. Talking to her helped them, too, as they processed the loss of their father.

Meanwhile, Jen joined a support group for widows and widowers. Not only did she make friends, but she was encouraged by listening to others who were navigating similar losses yet still able to thrive.

As she regained energy after the breast cancer treatments, she was able to volunteer at a co-op where families in need could get farm fresh produce. The friendships she formed at the co-op gave her a renewed sense of connection and joy. One day, a fellow volunteer invited Jen to a watercolor painting class. She'd never painted but soon fell in love with how she felt when painting. Painting became a source of creative expression and a way to celebrate the beauty of life.

Over the next five years, Jen began to reclaim joy. She painted vibrant coastal landscapes. One of her beachscapes is of where she and

Tim met and hangs in her home. For my fifty-fifth birthday, Jen gave me a painting of a sunrise over a choppy sea. The gray sea reminds me of all she's been through, while the sunrise reminds me of hope after loss.

At eighty, Jen's message to others is clear: Loss doesn't mean the end of joy. It's the beginning of a new kind of strength. I got to introduce Jen to my mother when she was eighty and Betty was ninety-two. At that meeting, Betty handed Jen a sheet of paper coiled up and wrapped in a ribbon. Betty gives this gift whenever someone loses a partner or is going through a divorce.

BETTY'S GIFT

These ideas helped me and may or may not help you. Either way, consider writing down your own learnings and passing them on to others who are going from being part of a couple to being solo.

1. Your sorrow (or happiness) is not your family's responsibility. They have lost a loved one, too.
2. When someone else has a loss, don't be shy about offering your friendship. Make an effort to help in their transition to single status.
3. Be an addition to a group—pick up the tab, be the driver, take your turn entertaining. Being a "victim" wears thin very fast.
4. Plan something. It is important to have "look forward" dates on your calendar.
5. Go out of your way to connect with others: Join a book club or an exercise group.
6. Put on a hat and sit outside reading in the sun. Watch TV until midnight if you choose!

> 7. Take someone else to a doctor's appointment and wait for them in the waiting room.
> 8. Explore your spirituality. "Blessed are those who mourn, for they shall be comforted."*
>
> ---
> * Matt. 5:4 (New King James Version)

RESILIENCE AND SPIRITUAL GROWTH

Resilience extends beyond mere survival. When our daughter, Claire, was diagnosed with a brain tumor at age twenty-four, a tidal wave of fear and grief crashed over her—and over me, her worried mother. It was an awful time, and the timing was terrible. Claire had been all packed for her move to attend medical school and become a doctor but found herself moving home to us to become a patient. As the neurosurgeons detailed the craniotomy, we tried to wrap our heads around possible deafness, facial paralysis, and the need to relearn how to walk. I felt the very real possibility of throwing up in the doctor's office from the weight of the information. Fortunately, I didn't get sick all over the office, but it was traumatic.

There is a phenomenon that psychologists call post-traumatic growth (PTG). PTG refers to the psychological changes and personal development that can occur as a result of struggling with highly challenging, stressful, or traumatic life events. Rather than being simply a return to baseline functioning, it involves surpassing previous levels of resilience, perspective, or well-being. Unexpectedly, our daughter's brain tumor and our associated trauma brought growth for me. I experienced spiritual growth, enabling me to develop a greater appreciation for life, stronger relationships, and a clearer recognition and acceptance that many things are out of our control. I had to face the fact that we can't protect our children from all the hard stuff. In a word, I'm more resilient because of what we went through. Claire, likewise, reports a greater empathy and a fiercer drive to help others. Survivors of traumatic illnesses often report feeling more connected to their values and a heightened sense of gratitude for life.[6] The transformative potential of hardship lies in its ability to deepen our connection to our core beliefs and values.

I am happy to report that Claire (and her brain tumor) are in medical school, as she and the neurosurgeons opted to "watch and wait" in hopes that the tumor will not grow. This circumstance, as well as the changing circumstances that will inevitably follow, are the building blocks of resilience. Resilience is more than enduring hardship; it's a catalyst for growth.

Regardless of what life brings, you can adapt with joy. Challenges will come, and while you can't predict the future, you can fortify your adaptability by using coping strategies, understanding grief, and recognizing the growth in resilience. You can experience joy all life long.

JOY PRACTICE:
You Are Resilient

In a journal or on a sheet of paper, write yourself a letter describing how you have grown through a challenge or a loss that you endured. End the letter with "You are resilient" because you are. The process of writing about a past situation can bolster you for current and future situations. Here is a letter I wrote to my former self about our daughter's brain tumor.

> *Dear Kerry of last year,*
> *I know you are surprised and scared about Claire's brain tumor. You cry a lot, especially by yourself in the garage. You feel sick that she is suffering and afraid. Here's the update: While she was so disappointed not to get to start the medical school*

she'd planned on attending, she just started at a different school even better suited to her interests and it's near her neurosurgeon. She opted to wait on the surgery and get MRIs every 6 months. Unlike how you feel now, in the future, you feel just fine, and so does Claire. You've grown spiritually and have greater maturity and humility. Anything can and will happen and you survived and will continue to survive when other things come your way. You got this, so come on out of the garage when you are ready. You are resilient.

Love,
Current Kerry

JOYSPANNER: Ruth Bader Ginsburg

Affectionately known as "RBG," Ruth Bader Ginsburg was a Supreme Court justice and a tireless advocate for gender equality. Despite facing significant obstacles throughout her life, she showed remarkable adaptability, resilience, and perseverance. Here are examples of why and how she had a long joyspan.

> **GROW:** Ginsburg was committed to lifelong learning and growth and continued her work as a Supreme Court justice into her eighties. Even after multiple battles with cancer, she maintained her rigorous work schedule, consistently delivering thoughtful and impactful rulings.
> **CONNECT:** She cultivated deep personal relationships, including her famously supportive marriage to Martin Ginsburg. Ruth was able to forge and maintain close friendships even across ideological divides (her friendship with Justice Antonin Scalia was well-known).

ADAPT: At Harvard Law School, she was one of nine women in a class of five hundred men. Hostile sex discrimination was part of her daily life. RBG found a way to succeed anyway. Further, when her husband and fellow student underwent treatment for testicular cancer in law school, Ruth attended classes as well as cared for their young daughter and her husband, all while excelling in her own studies. Upon graduation, when no law firm would hire a woman, she adapted her course to thrive even more, becoming a brilliant professor, relentless crusader for equality, and judge in the highest court in the land.

GIVE: RBG spent her life giving back through her legal work, creating pathways for women and marginalized communities. Her landmark cases and dissents continue to inspire generations to fight for equality and fairness in all aspects of life.

CHAPTER 7

Give with Joy

As I took the podium in a huge conference room at the Laguna Woods Village College Club in Southern California, the energy of the members was palpable. One hundred adults between the ages of 75 and 101 buzzed with intellectual curiosity. I opened the talk with a question: "What do you see as the purpose of these long lives?" I was glad I had on flat shoes because as people raised their hands, I had to speed walk with the cordless mic. An eighty-seven-year-old was the first to respond, saying, "The purpose of my long life is to share what I've learned with my grandchildren and great-grandchildren. What makes my life so meaningful is giving them all that I am."

The audience murmured in agreement, and to my delight, twenty more hands shot up. The next speaker said, "At eighty-two, my life is meaningful because of my friends, all widows. I'm bringing my leftovers from this luncheon to my friend Suellen because she's been sick. We care about one another, and we care for one another." Again, heads nodded.

Another attendee explained, "For eighty-nine years I've loved music. My great joy and purpose is sharing a beautiful piece of music with people who don't know music." Although each response was unique, together they reflected the fourth element of Joyspan: giving.

To give of yourself is to offer your time, energy, skills, or compassion to others, creating connections and fostering purpose. Giving is not just a moral ideal; it is an ongoing, action-based choice. Research shows that people who regularly give of themselves experience lower stress levels, better immune function, and increased life expectancy.[1] Giving reduces cortisol levels and activates neural pathways linked to reward and fulfillment.

Will Sharon's gift of time and energy to her grandchildren improve her well-being in longevity? Will Winnie's sharing of music enrich her Joyspan? The answer is a resounding yes. The science confirms it, as does the lived experience of thousands of people I've had the privilege of working with. Your purpose lies at the heart of giving.

YOUR PURPOSE IS TO GIVE

You can have a sense of purpose even if you can't readily recite, "My purpose is to...." Purpose exists in the small, everyday acts of care and contribution: nurturing relationships, sharing your passions, or contributing to your community.

Purpose is recognizing what you can give of yourself—and then giving it. It's a bridge connecting your inner values to the needs of others. You can have multiple giving intentions that wax and wane in importance over your lifetime as your priorities shift and your roles change. Purpose is a practice, and you create it and re-create it again and again. For example, a milestone birthday, retirement, divorce, or illness might make you reflect and reprioritize your purposes.

Recent research has provided evidence to support the idea that helping others goes hand in hand with meaningfulness. It's not just that people who have already found their purpose in life enjoy giving back. Instead, helping others can actually *create* the sense of meaning we're seeking. Rather than ruminating on what makes our life worthwhile as we work toward burnout, we can find the answer outside ourselves, in human connection.

Perhaps those who already feel like their lives have meaning are more motivated to help others, or perhaps some other factor (for example, spiritual beliefs) causes people to be helpful and experience more meaning in their lives. To examine this chicken-and-egg question, Daryl Van Tongeren and his colleagues asked more than four hundred participants to report on how frequently they engaged in giving behaviors (such as volunteering) and how meaningful their lives felt. Not surprisingly, participants who reported more giving behaviors reported a greater sense of purpose and meaning in their lives.[2]

Having a sense of purpose is a powerful predictor of all three aspects of longevity: lifespan, healthspan, and joyspan. Epidemiological research reveals that people with higher levels of life purpose have lower rates of cardiovascular disease, cognitive impairment, and all-cause mortality. What's more, having a stronger sense of purpose in life has been proved to impact how genes were expressed! Dr. Steven Cole and his team at UCLA collected DNA samples from 1,572 adults ages fifty to ninety-eight. They surveyed the participants on their self-reported level of happiness and self-reported level of life purpose. They were interested to see if self-reported happiness or level of life purpose impacted how genes were expressed.

The results were surprising—Dr. Cole said he was startled by the results. It was not how happy the participants felt that impacted gene expression, it was the extent to which people felt their lives had a sense of direction and purpose. The research showed that purpose caused lower inflammation and higher antiviral response. People with higher senses of purpose showed the opposite gene profile of those suffering from loneliness, who had elevated inflammation and reduced antiviral response, both of which increase disease processes.[3]

These findings have been repeated again and again. Lacking purpose can be as damaging as smoking or obesity. What a profound finding: Purpose is powerfully associated with well-being. Purpose transcends immediate self-gratification and connects people to something larger.

> "The only ones among you who will be really happy are those who have sought and found how to serve."
> —Albert Schweitzer

People who feel a sense of mission and engagement with life tend to also experience happiness. But not all the time. No one is happy all the time, and that is good and normal. Feeling like you have a reason to be—that's the biggie. Researcher Barbara Frederickson explains, "Purpose refers to those aspects of well-being that transcend immediate self-gratification and connect people to something larger."[4]

Another way to think about purpose is what Dr. Brian Little of Cambridge University calls "personal projects." He studied tens of thousands of these personal projects in thousands of research participants: things like training a dog, repairing a leak, sending birthday cards, tending a garden, being in a book club, looking in on a neighbor, and learning. He found that most people have around fifteen projects going at any one time.[5] To qualify, the projects must be meaningful to the person in some way. At their core, these projects all involve giving of yourself in a way that is meaningful to you.

Purpose Is Small

Let's say you now feel convinced by the research that increasing your sense of life purpose is worthwhile. How do you go about it? You don't need to begin with grand gestures; even small, everyday behaviors can have an impact on others and on your own sense of well-being. For example, in a study published in the journal *Science*, spending just five dollars on someone else led to boosts in happiness.[6] You can intentionally cultivate more kindness by writing down moments of kindness you observed, received, or gave at the end of each day.

Kindness and purpose are not big or loud gestures. For example, Lauren, a seventy-six-year-old neighbor, started small by baking cookies for her new neighbor, a young single dad. At first, Lauren thought it was just a nice gesture. But the simple act led to a heartfelt conversation, and Lauren discovered that her neighbor was struggling to balance work and childcare. Over the weeks, Lauren began offering to babysit for short periods, giving her neighbor much-needed breaks. In return, the young father taught Lauren how to use social media to stay connected with old friends. Through these small acts of kindness, Lauren not only felt a renewed sense of purpose but also built a meaningful friendship that brought joy to both their lives.

Purpose Is Kind

When you do something to make someone else's day brighter, that's kindness. Kindness comes in several flavors: compassion, generosity, empathy, selflessness, and warmth. But what does it really look like day-to-day? It can be small, almost invisible gestures or bigger acts of service. Kindness is as simple as holding the door open for a stranger whose arms are full or letting someone merge ahead of you in traffic with a smile instead of frustration. It's taking the time to compliment your spouse on their hard work or thanking a barista by name, even when you're in a rush. Sometimes, it's paying for the coffee of the person behind you in line, leaving a sticky note with a kind message on a doctor's desk, or offering to help your adult child who desperately needs a break from the kids.

On a more personal level, kindness can be about showing up. It's listening without judgment when a loved one needs to vent, texting a friend just to say you're thinking of them, or preparing a meal for someone going through a tough time.

What's remarkable isn't just that kindness is impactful in the moment—it's the fact that kindness is contagious. Research shows that witnessing or receiving kindness inspires others to pay it forward, creating a ripple effect. Psychologists call this "moral elevation," the warm, uplifting feeling we experience when we see someone being kind. This feeling makes us more likely to engage in kind acts ourselves. Individuals who observed acts of kindness were more likely to engage in prosocial behaviors themselves. One group of experiments revealed that participants who watched a video depicting generous actions donated 25 percent more to charity than those who viewed a neutral video.[7]

Imagine a work meeting where one person acknowledges the efforts of a team member. That small gesture tends to inspire others to do the same, fostering an environment of mutual respect. Or think of a busy subway platform where one person stops to help someone struggling with heavy bags. Suddenly, others nearby might step in to assist, shifting the mood of the crowd.

Kindness thrives in the mundane. It's the grocery clerk patiently helping an elderly shopper, a teacher pausing to give extra encouragement to a struggling student, or a neighbor shoveling snow from the walkway of the house next door. These everyday moments remind us that kindness is both accessible and transformative.

You usually don't realize how deeply your small acts affect others. A study from the University of Texas at Austin revealed that people underestimate the positive impact their kind actions have on others. This underestimation suggests that if individuals were more aware of the significant effects of their kindness, they might be more inclined to engage in such behaviors, thereby promoting a cycle of generosity.[8]

These findings underscore the powerful ripple effect that simple acts of kindness can have on your joyspan as well as the joyspan of others.

RATE YOUR SENSE OF PURPOSE

Take one minute to answer the four questions below to help you gauge where you are on fire with purpose or could put in a little more attention toward figuring it out.*

I am usually...
1. Bored
2. Slightly bored
3. Neither bored nor enthusiastic
4. Slightly enthusiastic
5. Enthusiastic

I know how I can use my talents to make a meaningful contribution to the larger world.
1. Strongly disagree
2. Disagree
3. Neither agree nor disagree
4. Agree
5. Strongly agree

How confident am I that I have discovered a satisfying purpose for my life?
1. Not at all
2. Slightly
3. Somewhat
4. Very
5. Extremely

---

* The questions are adapted and abbreviated from the Claremont Purpose Scale, the Purpose in Life Test, and the Life Engagement Test.

> *How much effort am I putting into making my goals a reality?*
> 1. Almost none
> 2. A little bit
> 3. Some
> 4. Quite a bit
> 5. A tremendous amount
>
> Adding the numbers you circled next to the responses above, your purpose score will fall between five and twenty-five. If your score is on the lower side of this range, you have a lower sense of purpose—right now. It is perfectly normal for one's sense of purpose to fluctuate over a lifetime. Attention to increasing your sense of purpose is likely all you need to boost it.

As you start thinking about clarifying your own sense of purpose, you may wonder whether it matters *what* you pursue. Research shows that the answer is yes—especially when you are older.

Life purpose groups comprise four categories:

Prosocial: This life purpose revolves around helping others, contributing to society, or making the world a better place. It focuses on altruism and the well-being of others. For example, a person who volunteers at a homeless shelter or starts a nonprofit organization to address climate change is living with a prosocial purpose.

Personal recognition: This purpose centers on achieving recognition, validation, or respect from others. It often involves striving for success, accomplishments, or leadership to gain admiration or prestige. For example, an athlete who trains tirelessly to win a gold medal or an artist who aims to have their work displayed in renowned galleries is driven by personal recognition.

Financial: This life purpose focuses on achieving financial stability, wealth, or material success. It often involves setting financial goals to improve one's quality of life or secure a legacy for future generations. For example, an entrepreneur building a business to generate wealth or a professional working toward early retirement is motivated by financial purpose.

Creative: This purpose is about expressing oneself, exploring ideas, or creating something unique and meaningful. It often involves innovation, artistry, or problem-solving. For example, a writer crafting a novel, a scientist conducting groundbreaking research, and a musician composing original songs are examples of those pursuing a creative purpose.

Each type of life purpose is distinct but can overlap with others, as individuals often find meaning in multiple categories simultaneously.

A longitudinal study looked at the relationship among the four types of purpose and well-being over time. The same group of participants were studied when they were young and again when they were older. When the sample was young, researchers didn't find differences in well-being according to the four purpose groups. It was just good to have a goal, no matter what it was. When the participants were older, those with prosocial purposes experienced significantly greater well-being.[9]

In a word, giving. Here are five ways to cultivate your sense of purpose by giving of yourself:

1. Cultivate giving.
2. Find what sparks you.
3. Brainstorm ways to use that spark.

4. Imagine the future you.
5. Try out some form of giving.

CULTIVATING GIVING

Last year I attended a memorial service for Gina Morgenson, my cherished friend who died from colon cancer. She left behind her husband and their three grown sons. Describing Gina, one sister said her purpose in life had been to *love without judgment.* A one-sentence mission statement I will always remember. Gina knew what she had to give—unconditional love—and she gave it freely every day. For example, Gina reached out to her friends and family members every day, regardless of how she felt or what treatment she was going through. She remembered what issues each of us was grappling with and would listen with such interest. You could tell Gina anything and never feel like she judged you for it; instead, she just loved you more for it.

After the service, a few of us stayed behind sharing memories of our Gina. Inspired by the impact of a life guided by loving without judgment, we thought about our own lives. At one friend's suggestion, we attempted brief purpose statements that could serve as guideposts for our lives. Here are our collective purpose statements:

- *To give my kids the financial and emotional security I never had*
- *To write poems to show others they are not alone*
- *To increase inclusion of people living with disabilities*
- *To improve the lives of older adults (that's mine)*
- *To bring joy to people by sharing my art*

None of us were certain we had it quite "right." All of us added the caveat that we "might change it later." When it comes to giving, there is no such thing as *right* or *final*. Life is always changing, needs are always changing, and we are always changing.

With these disclaimers in mind, if you were asked to come up with a sentence on your prosocial life purpose, what would it be? Here are four ideas to get the juices flowing.

Find What Sparks You

Begin by reflecting on what makes you feel alive—your passions and interests. Think about what you're good at, activities you enjoy, and values that are meaningful to you. Ask yourself, *What lights me up?* Your answers could range from family, nature, cooking, or social justice, to travel and beyond. Remember, your responses are as individual as you are, so allow yourself to roam freely and openly.

	Recognize What You Know	How to Give It to the World
What am I good at?	Listening Cooking Organizing	Visit homebound people. Organize a neighborhood get-together. Offer to help friends who feel overwhelmed.
What do I enjoy?	Teaching Reading Travel	Explore teaching options. Start a book club. Organize a group trip.
What matters to me?	Honoring God Eliminating the suffering of others	Find my way back to church. Join an organization aimed at addressing hunger, poverty, suicide, mental health problems, drug addiction, and loneliness.

Brainstorm Ways to Use That Spark

Once you've thought about what is meaningful to you, consider how you might give of yourself. My mother, Betty, uses her great listening skills and profound interest in others to provide invaluable support to friends and family. People of all ages call Betty when they have a victory to share or a problem weighing on them. Betty doesn't offer advice unless she's asked, but boy, she's got great ideas based on ninety-six years of experience. Whenever I call her and get a busy signal, I know she's helping someone.

> "It was only a sunny smile, and little it cost in the giving; but it scattered the night like morning light."
> —F. Scott Fitzgerald

If You Had a Wand That Worked

If you woke up tomorrow and found yourself with the power to immediately change two things, what would you change? Let's say your two changes were: (1) eradicating world hunger; and (2) helping the young single mother next door to pay her rent. Ask yourself why you chose those two options. You might gain insight on what matters to you and what kind of giving you would like to pursue.

Imagine the Future You

Think of yourself at some older age. For example, if you are seventy, picture yourself at age ninety. Imagine this future you as the best possible version—radiant, healthy, engaged, connected, and beloved. What are you doing? What is important to you? Who are you with?

What do you care about and why? Now take it even further and imagine that ideal future self has passed away after a long, rich life. What are they saying at your funeral? To maximize the benefit of this exercise, write out your answer. To make it even more powerful, read what you wrote out loud. In doing this, you are clarifying what is meaningful to you and you are on your way to becoming that version of yourself.

Try Out Some Form of Giving

Sample some things you might enjoy by giving them a shot. Do you have an inkling that you are interested in animals? Head over to your local animal shelter and either just spend time with the animals or check on a volunteer or paid position. Maybe it will become clear that it is not for you, and you can cross it off the list. Or perhaps you have an inner Dr. Dolittle and will feel your sense of purpose soar. Don't put any pressure on your explorations. You are simply dipping your toe into the water to see if the temperature is right before you plunge in. This approach also puts you in touch with people who may inspire you or suggest other opportunities for making a difference that you hadn't thought of before.

GIVING GOALS

My brother, Russ, enjoyed a long career in real estate and recently retired. After the novelty of "no schedule" wore off, he started to feel uncomfortable. After sixty-four years of giving—at work, and with his three kids—where did he fit in now? One day, he stood behind a young mother and her five-year-old son in the supermarket. The boy had an endless string of questions for his exhausted mother, still in her work uniform. "Hey, Mom, what's hummus? How many cookies are in that box? What flavor is yellow?"

Russ recalled those days when he was a young parent thirty years earlier. As the little boy continued his onslaught of questions, he wished he could somehow help the boy's mother. Just as he was pondering the question, the boy said, "Hey, Mom, Mrs. Picciano is sick, so we had a substitute teacher; she's called a sub. Mom, have you ever had a sub?"

Struck with inspiration, Russ researched what it would take to become a substitute teacher and found that there was a significant shortage in his community. Further, in the substitute pool there were hardly any men. So Russ went through the trainings, background checks, and requirements. His first assignment was filling in for a kindergarten teacher. He was nervous and wondered if this was a good idea, having never taught school. Would he have the stamina?

He walked into a packed room filled with wide eyes. "Good morning, boys and girls. I'm Mr. Russ," he announced. A bold boy asked, "Are you old?" The classroom fell to a hush as all the children zeroed in on the sub. With a big grin, he replied, "I have gray hair and glasses, so that's a great guess! I am old compared to you, and young compared to others." The children were thrilled. They went home to their parents with stories of fun, older Mr. Russ.

Soon all the kindergarten teachers were requesting him as their substitute. Over time, Russ became close friends with the other teachers, the principal, the office staff, the yard monitors, and the parents. Russ was able to select the days he worked. A few months into the job, his dermatologist diagnosed him with skin cancer, an occupational hazard for surfers like himself.

The surgery to remove the carcinoma left a gaping scar on his forehead. Rather than hide the scar, Mr. Russ played it up upon his return. With great fanfare and a wand, he reintroduced himself to the kindergartners as Mr. Harry Potter. The kids were over the moon, and Russ is setting himself up to enjoy a joyspan as long as his lifespan. Proud sister here (see figure 12).

FIGURE 12. Joyspan Matrix in Action: Russ, Age 67

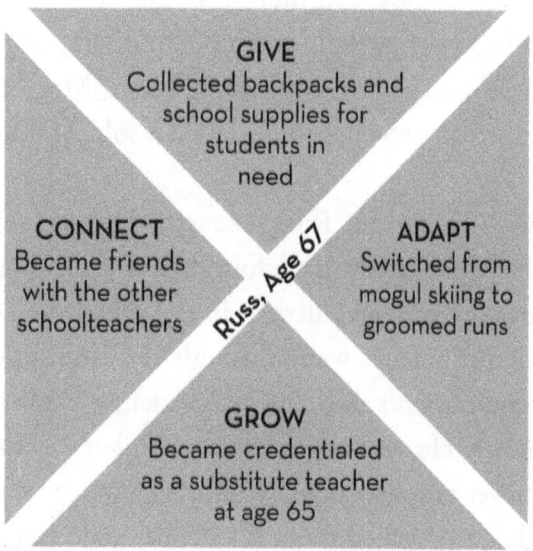

What are your giving goals? Like Russ, are you interested in giving back to the community? Or maybe your giving goals lie in a more spiritual realm? For example, Angie often found herself reflecting on life's uncertainties after her husband passed away. She began walking daily through a nearby forest, where she felt a connection to something greater. As the seasons changed around her—buds in spring, leaves falling in autumn—Angie saw parallels to her own life's transitions. Her spiritual connection to the natural world gave her a profound sense of peace and meaning. This practice didn't erase her grief, but it helped her embrace life's challenges with a renewed sense of purpose and spiritual clarity.

In a similar way, James, an eighty-one-year-old retired firefighter, had always considered himself a man of action, not reflection. But as he faced macular degeneration, he started feeling untethered, questioning his purpose now that his career and daily responsibilities had ended. One evening, while sorting through old belongings, he stumbled upon a worn Bible his mother had given him years ago. He opened it to a verse in the Book of Psalms she had underlined: *"Be still, and know that I am God."*[10]

Inspired, James began setting aside time each morning to sit quietly with the Bible, reflecting on its messages and writing down his thoughts. Over time, this ritual became a source of grounding and clarity. Through this spiritual practice, he came to see his life's challenges as part of a larger story, and he found new ways to serve others—mentoring younger firefighters and volunteering at his local church. His sense of purpose deepened, and his days felt imbued with peace and meaning.

In addition to community goals and spiritual goals, is it possible that your giving goals involve mentorship? One of the most profound ways to make sense of your life is by sharing your journey with others. Offer your experiences and lessons to younger generations or peers through mentorship, storytelling, or volunteering to teach a skill you've mastered. By giving your wisdom to others, you gain clarity on how your experiences fit together and provide valuable guidance to those who may benefit from your insights.

Trin, a seventy-year-old retired nurse, felt a growing sense of restlessness after leaving the profession she loved. She volunteered at the hospital and shared lunch breaks with nurses who were early in their careers. When they asked about her thirty-two years in practice, Trin began to see her own life in a new light—her years of hard work, perseverance, and compassion became a narrative of resilience and purpose. On her birthday, she got a note from one of the nurses that read "I was wondering if I could handle being a mom and being a nurse, and seeing how you did it made me realize that I can, too."

Goals provide direction, energy, and fulfillment. Goals help you wake up and hit the ground running. Another way to clarify your giving goals is to revisit former goals. Every life is littered with goals that have been cast aside for various reasons. Were you too busy to paint? Too broke to travel? Too shy to try your hand at stand-up comedy? Now is the time to try to remember, and reconsider, old goals. Far too many lives end before fulfilling the dreams they've held in secret while waiting for the right time. The time to pursue long-held dreams? Right now.

> "Often the best and easiest way to improve your own sense of meaningfulness is to switch your lens: Concentrate less on yourself and more on being connected with others."
> —Frank Martela, Finnish philosopher and researcher

JOY PRACTICE:
Give of the Day

Every morning, take a moment to reflect on how you can give something meaningful to someone else. Ask yourself:

- Who could use a kind gesture today?
- What small act of generosity can I offer?
- How can I contribute to someone's well-being or happiness?

Choose your give. Your act of giving can be as simple or creative as you like. Here are examples:

- **Tangible gift:** Surprise someone with their favorite coffee, bake a treat to share, or leave a thoughtful note.
- **Emotional support:** Reach out to someone who may be struggling and offer a listening ear or encouraging words.
- **Acts of kindness:** Hold the door open, compliment a stranger, or help someone with a task.
- **Time or presence:** Dedicate uninterrupted time to a loved one, free from distractions. This is different from emotional support in that it can be done in silence. It is the gift of just being present.

Perform your "Give of the Day" with intention and without expectation of recognition or something in return. Focus on the positive energy you are creating for both yourself and others. At the end of the day, take a moment to reflect on how your act of giving made you feel. Do you think it brought someone any joy? Did it bring you any joy?

Why It Works:

- **Giving boosts joy:** Giving activates neural pathways associated with happiness and fulfillment, often referred to as the "giver's high."
- **Giving fosters connection:** Small acts of giving build and strengthen relationships, reminding you of your significance to others.
- **Giving creates purpose:** Daily generosity reinforces a sense of purpose and contribution, helping you live each day with meaning.

Example in practice: Colleen, a mother who struggled to find purpose after her four children left home, decided to implement the "Give of the Day" practice. One day, she baked cookies and delivered them to an older neighbor who had recently lost her husband. Another day, she spent an hour helping a young mother at the park who was overwhelmed with her toddler. Each tiny act left Colleen feeling more connected to her community and gave her a sense of fulfillment that brightened her days.

Challenge: For the next seven days, commit to practicing "Give of the Day" and notice how it transforms your mood, your relationships, and your overall sense of joy and purpose. Giving has the power to make every day more meaningful.

Another Example in Practice

Meet Joanna. After retiring from her long and successful career in marketing and watching her two children move across the country, her once-busy days were now quiet. She spent her mornings scrolling through social media, comparing her mundane life to the (seemingly) adventurous lives of others. The more she focused on herself—what she lacked, what she'd lost—the deeper her feelings of insignificance grew. Joanna researched opportunities to give and found a food bank.

At the pantry, Joanna met a young single father named Marcus, who was juggling a job and raising two small children. Jo listened intently as he shared his struggles. For the first time in a long while, her focus shifted outward. She began to notice other faces at the pantry—an older woman who had recently lost her husband; a young man new to the city and searching for work.

Joanna didn't just help hand out groceries; she started talking to the people she met, learning their stories. She realized that while she couldn't solve all their problems, her kindness—offering a warm smile, a listening ear, or an encouraging word—made a real difference.

As weeks turned into months, Jo began taking on more responsibility at the pantry, organizing donation drives and mentoring younger volunteers. She discovered that her marketing skills, which she once believed were irrelevant, would be invaluable in creating campaigns that brought in much-needed support for the pantry.

Through giving of what she had, Joanna regained her sense of purpose. She no longer spent her days thinking about what she'd lost but focused on what she could give.

Joanna showed me a handwritten note she'd received from Marcus: "Quick note to tell you I got the job at Enterprise Car Rental like you suggested. Thank you for believing in me because I wasn't really believing in myself." By shifting her focus outward, Joanna found a renewed sense of purpose and meaning. Often, giving to others is the greatest gift we can give ourselves.

CONCLUSION: YOUR JOYSPAN LEGACY

One of my most treasured possessions is a small, tattered notepad that belonged to my grandmother Charlotte. The cover is worn, and the pages are filled with shaky, uneven cursive—short notes she had written to herself in the final months of her life. The entries seem mundane at first glance: "Evening News at 5 p.m." jotted in one corner, a circled $4.11 toward the bottom, and a note about "Betty emery boards" on the lower left. Yet, on one page, she had copied an Eleanor Roosevelt quote, which was the reason the notepad escaped the waste bin and became an heirloom. The words read:

> When you cease to make a contribution,
>   you begin to die.
> The purpose of life is to live it,
> to taste experience to the utmost,
> to reach out eagerly and without fear
> for newer and richer experience.
> —E. Roosevelt

At that stage in her life, just weeks before her passing, writing wasn't easy for Charlotte, but the First Lady's words struck her deeply enough that she made the effort. They encapsulated how she lived her life and the values she passed on to those who came after her. Charlotte embraced herself as an older person, refusing to let age diminish her ability to give, to find purpose, and to experience joy. Charlotte enjoyed a long joyspan, and her example was a gift. Her legacy lives on in her daughter, Betty, who at ninety-six continues to embody those same ideals. Betty, too, has become a role model, showing that aging is not all decline but a chapter rich with meaning.

For too long, society has viewed older life as a period of loss and limitation. But Charlotte's notepad reminds us of a profound truth: Growing older can be a time of contribution, growth, and joy. Every choice you make today, every act of generosity, contributes to your joyspan.

Your joyspan legacy challenges the narrative of aging and redefines it. By embracing aging as a time to give of yourself, to live with purpose, and to experience joy, you set an example for those who follow you.

Eleanor Roosevelt's words ripple outward. Charlotte's example shaped Betty's life, and Betty's life continues to shape those around her. Your joyspan will inspire your children, grandchildren, and even strangers to view aging not as an ending but as a rich and vital continuation—a time to live fully and give generously. Maximize your joyspan legacy by asking yourself:

- *What do I have to give?* Reflect on your interests and resources. The world needs what you have to offer, whether it's wisdom, time, skills, kindness, or even regular smiles at people you encounter. Small, intentional acts offered with love create a lasting impact.
- *How can I give with purpose today?* Purpose is what gives life meaning at every stage. It's found in the ways you connect with others, the passions you pursue, and the values you embody. Purpose evolves as you evolve.
- *What creates moments of joy for me, and how might I share it with others?* Joy is contagious: savoring the smell of a pine tree, a funky antique market, fostering pets, a Harley-Davidson motorcycle, an invitation to tea. Find what lights you up and share it with the people you know, and the people you don't know—yet.

Together, we can change the narrative around aging. Charlotte's life—and her small notepad—reminds us that our contributions add up. We can turn the world into one in which aging is celebrated as a time to create, to mentor, and to give of our authentic selves. The purpose of life is to live it—with as much joy as you can muster.

JOYSPANNER: Albert Schweitzer

Albert Schweitzer was a scholar nearing middle age, with doctorates in theology, philosophy, music, and medicine, when he decided to go "all in" with giving. He went to the interior of Africa to give of himself in hopes of bringing healing to people who didn't have access to medical care. He brought with him a piano wrapped in a zinc case so he could play Bach in the evenings for his patients and colleagues. Amid the cicadas and snakes, music and healing permeated the village. Despite the decades of danger he faced, Albert Schweitzer had a joyspan equal to his lifespan, ninety years.

- **GROW:** The second half of Albert's life was the time of his greatest growth—by far. When most of his colleagues were winding down their medical careers, Albert was just getting started. He didn't know if he could achieve his goal of serving people in need in a foreign land, but he pushed himself to go for it anyway. He tried, and often that is all the difference.
- **CONNECT:** He cultivated deep relationships with his patients and colleagues in Africa. He was a serious and at times demanding man, but those who worked with him related that under his walrus mustache and furrowed forehead, there was warmth, friendship, and caring.

ADAPT: Despite limited resources, skepticism, and an array of overwhelming daily challenges, Schweitzer continuously adapted as a person in order to meet the evolving needs of his community and mission. He adjusted his approach to balance medical care with cultural sensitivity and respect. As he grew older and had less energy, he adapted his practice so he could use his diminishing energy wisely, doling it out thoughtfully to maximize his service.

GIVE: Dr. Schweitzer's giving was characterized by astounding risk and self-sacrifice. When he arrived in Africa in 1913, 75 percent of the inhabitants in a nearby village died in one year under a single wave of sleeping sickness. He knew he was risking his life in making the leap and he dived in anyway.

PART III

How to Create Your Joyspan

CHAPTER 8

Filling Your Joytank

Welcome to part 3 of this book. Here you'll find the essential tools and insights to help you sustain your joyspan. You'll discover how to fill your joytank by harnessing the unique strengths and opportunities that come with aging. This section will also cover what to do when your joyspan dips, offering practical strategies to reignite your sense of purpose and fulfillment. Most importantly, you'll learn how to make every moment of your joyspan count, ensuring that your later years are not just long, but long and joy-filled.

In graduate school, I fell in love with the work of a neurologist named Dr. Oliver Sacks. In his book *The Man Who Mistook His Wife for a Hat*, Dr. Sacks introduced me to patients living with baffling neurological conditions. His patients Michael and John were twins who could easily memorize a string of numbers of three hundred digits but couldn't manage basic self-care. Jimmie G. suffered from acute amnesia, lost thirty years' worth of memories, and was unable to recall anything for more than a minute. Dr. P. was a music teacher whose perceptual abilities were so impaired that he thought his wife's head was his hat.

As I read these case histories, I was struck by the complexity of the brain and by the loving way Dr. Sacks wrote about his patients. He honored the innate dignity and value of each patient, an approach so different from the cold medical culture I'd worked in up to that point. Over the course of my career, I read all of Dr. Sacks's books, and he influenced my work with older adults living with memory differences.

Over the years I followed his career and got to observe how he applied his humanistic principles to his own aging. He welcomed and celebrated growing older and all that came with it. In an article about turning eighty, he described how he saw older age not as a shrinking but as an enlargement of mental life and perspective. He found his later decades to be some of the most enjoyable years of his life. Dr. Sacks intentionally created his joyspan.

> "I do not think of old age as an ever-grimmer time that one must somehow endure and make the best of, but as a time of freedom, freed from the factitious urgencies of earlier days, free to explore whatever I wish, and to bind the thoughts and feelings of a lifetime together."
>
> —*Oliver Sacks*

Ten years ago, I was at the breakfast table reading the *New York Times* when I jolted to attention after noticing an op-ed by Dr. Sacks titled "My Own Life." He was then eighty-one and swimming a mile a day. The piece started with, "My luck has run out—a few weeks ago I learned that I have multiple metastases in the liver." My heart sank but was comforted and not surprised that Dr. Sacks greeted his diagnosis with his characteristic thoughtfulness and zest for life. He described how the news gave him a deepening sense of connection to life. He explained, "It does not mean I am finished with life. On the contrary, I feel intensely alive, and I want and hope in the time that remains to deepen my friendships, to say farewell to those I love, to write more, to travel if I have the strength, to achieve new levels of understanding and insight." Talk about joyspan all the way to the end!

How did Dr. Sacks navigate aging and death with joy? How do you and I? Dr. Sacks capitalized on what gets better as you get older to maximize joy and meaning. He paid attention to how he was feeling and made small tweaks to his daily life to keep his spirits up. He kept tabs on his mindset about his own aging.

This chapter shows you how to fill your joytank by

- using what gets better as you get older;
- paying attention to your emotional well-being;
- making tweaks to your emotional well-being; and
- checking in on your aging beliefs using the Joyspan Grid.

USE WHAT GETS BETTER AS YOU GET OLDER TO MAXIMIZE JOY

When you think about aging, what jumps to mind? Diminished stamina, reduced speed, lost collagen? With all the emphasis on what's lost, a crucial part of the conversation has been missing: what gets better as you get older. A growing body of research shows that aging also brings gains, qualities that deepen over time. Of the many strengths that you gain with age, let's focus upon five:

1. You don't care as much what others think of you.
2. You enjoy greater emotional stability.
3. You draw upon experience-based problem-solving.
4. You explore greater depth of spirituality.
5. You choose to laugh.

Why haven't you heard about these? The "antiaging industry" has done a fantastic job of convincing you that it's all downhill. In lamenting what gets worse, you've missed what gets better. As younger people, many of us thought we were superior to older folks in every way. Nope. In some areas, we are stronger as we get older.

> "My secret at ninety-six? Play to your strengths. Compared to when I was young, I'm more even-keeled, less of a people pleaser. I laugh at things that used to send me. I'm a more thoughtful friend."
> —Betty Parker, my mother

Not recognizing and capitalizing upon what gets better as you get older is like floating down the river of life without realizing that you have an oar—and not just one oar but a group of oars that are powerful in different situations.

YOU DON'T CARE AS MUCH WHAT OTHERS THINK OF YOU

Four words that may have single-handedly stopped you from trying something new, singing out loud, pursuing a dream, and taking a chance: *What would people think?* In the younger years, the "disease to please" often has us jumping through hoops and catering to the opinions of others. Needing to be liked by everyone is not only exhausting, it's impossible.

People pleasers, take heart. Concern over others' opinions decreases significantly after age fifty. Adults experience a reduced reliance on external validation and are less likely to dwell on social judgments.[1] Why is this? First, neurological changes in the brain play a role. We have reduced activity in the medial prefrontal cortex, which is the part of the brain involved with social evaluation. Second, with a lifetime of experiences, we understand that we will never please everyone. We aren't devastated if someone disagrees or disapproves. In fact, we may not even care.

This shift from self-consciousness to self-confidence is one of the liberating gifts of growing older. As a younger woman, J. K. Rowling was deeply self-conscious. She worried constantly about how others perceived her, doubted her writing ability, and feared judgment. These insecurities nearly kept her from pursuing her dreams. As she grew older, the judgment of others began to hold less sway over her. She learned to separate her self-worth from external validation, which gave her the courage to submit her manuscript—and thank heaven she did.

> "It is impossible to live without failing at something
> unless you live so cautiously that you
> might as well not have lived at all—in
> which case, you fail by default."
>
> —*J. K. Rowling*

After many rejections, Rowling got a publisher to take a chance on her. Had she remained shackled to the opinions of others, the brilliant Harry Potter books would be a dusty stack of paper on a shelf. It is hard to get anything done while wearing the handcuffs of caring what people will think. Not caring as much what people think about you allows you to live more authentically, unapologetically, and joyfully. When you use this strength of older age, you experience:

- **Greater confidence:** It's easier to express yourself authentically without fear of judgment.
- **Improved mental health:** Reduced social anxiety strengthens emotional well-being.
- **Stronger relationships:** Genuine connections flourish when you are less preoccupied with maintaining appearances.
- **Increased focus on personal goals:** By letting go of external expectations, you can dedicate energy to your passions and aspirations.

Not everyone enjoys a reduction in how much they care about what others think of them as they age. If you were raised in an environment that emphasized appearances and external validation, it may be especially hard, but take heart, you, too, can free yourself. Pursuing intrinsic goals successfully reduces the need for external validation.[2]

Here's how to pursue intrinsic goals to set yourself free:

1. Identify what truly matters to you—things like spending time with loved ones, pursuing hobbies, or contributing to your community—and focus your energy there.
2. Regularly reflect on whether your actions align with your personal values rather than societal expectations.
3. Set goals that prioritize fulfillment and joy over external validation, such as trying something new or improving a skill for your own satisfaction.

YOU ENJOY GREATER EMOTIONAL STABILITY

Maya Angelou's childhood trauma led her to stop speaking for nearly five years. She grew up amid racial discrimination, poverty, and personal hardships, including becoming a single mother at age seventeen.

Throughout her early adulthood, Angelou navigated a turbulent life, working a variety of jobs and moving across continents. She felt adrift and emotionally unstable.

Even with all the cards stacked against her, as Angelou grew older, her perspective on life and her emotional stability began to shift. She found solace in writing, using it as a tool to process her experiences and connect with others. In middle age she published her groundbreaking autobiography, *I Know Why the Caged Bird Sings*, which allowed her to reflect on her past with greater understanding and compassion. Angelou credited her greater emotional stability to getting older and to deciding to forgive (see figure 13).

> "You may not control all the events that happen to you, but you can decide not to be reduced by them."
> —*Maya Angelou*

FIGURE 13. Joyspan Matrix in Action: Maya Angelou, Age 86

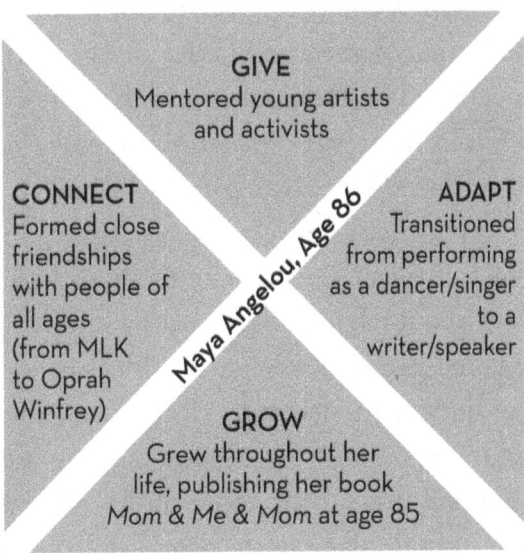

Growing older is linked to greater emotional stability and overall well-being. A study from the Stanford Center on Longevity showed that older people are more emotionally balanced, can better solve emotional problems, and are more adept at resisting emotional temptations, such as lashing out in anger or becoming overly disturbed by setbacks.[3]

One explanation lies in changes to the amygdala, the brain's emotional processing center. As we age, the amygdala becomes less reactive to negative stimuli, helping us maintain a calm and composed demeanor. Combined with years of experience in navigating life's ups and downs, this makes older adults more emotionally resilient.

YOU DRAW UPON EXPERIENCE-BASED PROBLEM-SOLVING

When it comes to our brains and aging, a lot of the news isn't great. Studies show age-associated declines in processing speed, working memory, executive functions, and language. These changes are the result of slowing nerve impulses and atrophy in the cerebral cortex.

Fortunately, when it comes to your brain, it is not all downhill. There is an important cognitive ability that can get better as you grow older: experience-based problem-solving. It draws upon accumulated knowledge and skills from past experiences to resolve new challenges. It is grounded in *crystallized intelligence*—the ability to use learned knowledge and experience to solve problems. This contrasts with *fluid intelligence*, which involves the capacity to think logically and solve novel problems without relying on preexisting knowledge.

Experience-based problem-solving is critical in scenarios requiring on-the-spot judgment decisions. Remember the grandparents stranded at the train station from chapter 6? They used their strong experience-based problem-solving ability to have a pizza delivered to their son's home and ride along in the pizza delivery car.

When you've lived long enough, you start to see patterns in life. Most problems aren't new—they're just new to the person facing them. When I was a young professor, a pipe burst at the university. We sloshed about while the water in our offices steadily rose. With a calm nonchalance, Dr. White, our eighty-year-old colleague, quietly shut off the water and then handed out towels to each of us, her drowned-rat-looking colleagues.

Are you capitalizing on your experience-based problem-solving abilities? The next time you face a challenge, take a moment to reflect on similar situations you've handled in the past. What worked? What didn't? Draw on your own "solution playbook" to help you navigate current obstacles with greater confidence and efficiency.

YOU EXPLORE GREATER DEPTH OF SPIRITUALITY

Despite growing up in a Jewish home, Oliver Sacks was neither religious nor spiritual as a younger person because he felt alienated from organized religion. When he was eighteen, his father pushed him to discuss his romantic interests, asking if he liked males rather than females. "I haven't *done* anything," young Oliver said. "It's just a feeling—but don't tell Ma; she won't be able to take it." His father did tell his mother, and the next morning she confronted him with a look of horror on her face and shrieked: "You are an abomination. I wish you had never been born." The matter was never mentioned again, but her harsh words made him hate religion's capacity for cruelty.

With age, Dr. Sacks grew into a spiritual man devoted to learning what is meant by living a good and worthwhile life. Toward the end of his life, he also became more religious and wrote about the meaning of the Sabbath in Judaism.

Consider your spiritual life: Do you think about the meaning of life? Do you consider yourself a religious person? In the World Values Survey, researchers asked two questions of 86,274 people in sixty countries. The first question was a rough proxy measure of spirituality and the second of religiosity. Here's what they found: Of the polled people, 64 percent said they were religious and 78 percent said they were spiritual.[4] This was the average; results on the religion question varied widely, with only 13 percent of respondents in China saying they were religious, compared to 97 percent of respondents in Nigeria. There was much more consistency about spirituality: In every country, 51 to 92 percent of respondents said they thought about spirituality.

What about differences by age? Older respondents rated themselves as more religious and more spiritual than did younger respondents. If you are wondering whether this difference is because we become more spiritual or religious as we age or because of generational issues, it's both. With age, people tend to seek meaning and reflect on their life experiences; also, older cohorts often grew up in more religiously oriented societal contexts, shaping their lifelong beliefs and practices.[5]

Greater depth in spirituality and religion improves lifespan, healthspan, and joyspan. Studies from around the world show that those who report religious or spiritual practices have:

- **Longer life expectancy:** a four- to seven-year increase in life expectancy, depending on practice[6]
- **Improved physical health:** lower blood pressure, lower cholesterol, less heart disease and stroke
- **Improved mental health:** lower rates of depression and anxiety
- **Stronger social connections:** higher social support and greater companionship
- **Enhanced coping mechanisms:** increased tools for coping with loss, grief, and life changes

Spiritual life and religious life can improve as you get older and are very good for your physical and mental health. How do you expand your spiritual experience in older age? Pope Francis taught that one way to grow spiritually in older age is to shift how you view yourself. Rather than see yourself as the flower on a tree, or even the trunk of a tree, see yourself as the root of the tree. The root system is essential for holding up the flowers, branches, and trunk.[7] As roots, the thing we can always do, no matter how old or frail we become, is love. As the current matriarchs and patriarchs of society, we can love more fiercely than ever. We can pass on history, faith, and love to the coming generations. We can be role models of the internal beauty of advancing years. We can change the narrative around aging.

When you draw upon your spiritual strengths, gifts such as wisdom, love, and gratitude, you have so much to offer the world. As you get older, you see that life is gray rather than black-and-white. In an interview with British researcher Jane Kuepfer, an eighty-year-old explained, "My faith today is stronger than it would have been any time throughout my life, but I question more things than I would ever have questioned. When I was twenty-five years old, my faith would have been very black-and-white. Today I'm not as sure about many things. Most people would look at that as saying my faith is weakened, but I think my faith is stronger."[8]

By drawing upon faith, we grow not only as people, but also in our ability to inspire and assist in the faith development of future generations.

YOU CHOOSE TO LAUGH

My colleague Lee had a parrot named Tony. To Lee's delight, Tony learned to say, "Hello, pretty birdie." Unfortunately, Tony also learned insults, complete with swear words. Lee tried everything to reform the parrot—playing classical music, using positive reinforcement, even reading motivational quotes aloud. But nothing worked.

One day, after the parrot called Lee a "lazy @#%*" in front of his mother-in-law, Lee lost his patience. "That's it!" he yelled. "You're going in the freezer to cool off!"

He gently placed the parrot in the freezer, thinking a short time-out might teach it a lesson. For the first few seconds, the parrot squawked and screeched, clearly outraged. Then, suddenly, silence.

Worried he'd gone too far, Lee flung open the freezer door. The parrot calmly walked out, shivering slightly but looking oddly serene. "I sincerely apologize for my behavior," it said. "I now understand the error of my ways and will strive to be a polite and courteous parrot moving forward."

Lee was stunned. "Well...I'm glad we're on the same page," he said.

The parrot nodded solemnly, then glanced back at the freezer. "By the way," it asked quietly, "may I ask, what exactly did the chicken do?"

This anecdote about Lee was from a ninety-two-year-old friend named Gawky, who always had a joke ready for me.

Did you know that your sense of humor can and often does get better as you get older? This is good news because laughter reduces stress, boosts the immune system, and even improves pain tolerance. Freed from the self-consciousness of youth, many people find it easier to laugh at life's absurdities and at themselves. Why does humor get better with age?

EXPERIENCE PROVIDES PERSPECTIVE

Life's ups and downs teach us that most challenges are temporary, and many are beautifully absurd in hindsight. A missed bus, a spilled glass of red wine, or an embarrassing faux pas can transform from stressful to hilarious with time and perspective when you laugh at yourself.

> "If you can laugh at yourself, you'll never run out of material."
>
> —John Parker, my dad (who laughed a lot)

EMOTIONAL REGULATION IMPROVES

As you age, your ability to regulate emotions strengthens. Instead of reacting with anger or frustration, you are more likely to laugh things off. This shift is linked to the brain's growing preference for positive emotional experiences.

WISDOM AND RELATABILITY

You are more likely to embrace imperfections and see the humor in the human condition. You've lived through enough to realize that life is often unpredictable and ridiculous— and that's a good thing.

SOCIAL CONNECTION THROUGH HUMOR

Laughter fosters bonds, and you can use humor to maintain relationships. This is particularly true when sharing stories of your misadventures, which can turn mundane life events into comedic gold.

STAY AWARE OF YOUR JOYSPAN

Joyspan in longevity is a dynamic and ongoing process. To nurture it, it's important to keep tabs on your feelings, make adjustments as needed, and approach challenges with curiosity and resilience.

Tracking how you feel isn't just about identifying big emotions—it's about noticing subtle shifts and responding proactively.

The butterfly effect, a concept from chaos theory, suggests that small actions or changes can create ripple effects leading to profound outcomes. The term comes from meteorologist Edward Lorenz, who proposed that the flap of a butterfly's wings in Brazil could set off a tornado in Texas, illustrating how tiny, seemingly unrelated factors can have massive impacts over time.[9]

In the context of your joyspan, even the smallest positive adjustments—such as a five-minute stretch, a kind word, or a new way of thinking—can cascade into meaningful improvements in your overall quality of life. For example, a walk can inspire you to tackle larger health goals; a text can reignite a relationship; and writing a few sentences in a journal can clarify your thoughts. Small changes seem insignificant in isolation, but over time, they compound to maximize joy and well-being in longevity.

Now that you understand the ways in which life can improve as you age, here are some tools to help make sure you capitalize upon what gets better as you get older. Too often, people inadvertently start living their lives on autopilot as they age. Avoid this! As you grow older you need more self-awareness and course corrections than ever to navigate the increasingly challenging terrain of life.

DAILY CHECK-IN HABIT

Establish a consistent time each day to "check in" with yourself. This practice creates a moment of mindfulness, allowing you to better understand your emotional, physical, and mental states.

Questions to ask yourself:

How do I feel physically? (Energetic, tired, achy?)
How do I feel mentally? (Foggy, sharp, organized, confused?)

How do I feel emotionally? (Content, stressed, sad, excited?)
What brought me joy today? (Even the smallest moments count.)

For many people, journaling enhances the check-in process by helping them track patterns over time. Write at least a few sentences each day about what you are grateful for, how you are feeling, and your goals. Look for trends. If Mondays are always gloomy, you might schedule a lunch date with a friend or start the week with a small treat to lift your spirits.

In his memoir *On the Move*, Oliver Sacks describes his daily habit of reflecting while swimming laps. He checked in with himself and took the time to focus upon moments of joy—a look on a patient's face, a moment of music, time on his motorcycle, a sunset. Similarly, Betty finds she feels more grounded on days she takes five minutes to list a few things she is grateful for. This simple practice helps her to reframe challenges and to approach her day with more optimism.

MAKE NEEDED TWEAKS

When you regularly check in with yourself, you'll be able to identify when it's time to make adjustments. The "tweak" that needs to be made will be different for everyone. In your journal, create a list of physical, mental, and emotional tweaks that you can use as a menu when you feel off. The list below is an example. Your list will be longer and specifically tailored to what works for you.

Physical tweaks: When you notice you are feeling tired, achy, or low on energy:

- Take a ten-minute walk.
- Drink an extra glass of water each day.

- Stretch at home or in a yoga or stretch class.
- Have a nutritious snack like some quality protein, fiber, or other unprocessed food.

Mental tweaks: When your mind feels foggy, scattered, or overwhelmed:

- Increase your physical activity.
- Take steps to improve the quality and amount of your sleep.
- Check your medications and their side effects.
- Reduce or eliminate alcohol intake.

Emotional tweaks: When you feel down, empty, or disconnected:

- Text, call, or write a letter, with no agenda, to someone—just to connect.
- Swap a passive activity (like watching TV) for something active, such as reading, painting, or gardening.
- Do a random act of kindness.
- Turn on some music and sing your heart out.

Joy tweaks: When you aren't sure what the problem is, and you just feel blah:

- Create a list of things that bring you joy.
- Go outside and take in nature.
- Watch a favorite comedy or read a funny book.
- Schedule time for a hobby that makes you lose track of time.
- Try something new—like cooking a new dish or visiting a new museum.

REVIEW YOUR JOYSPAN GRID EVERY SO OFTEN

What you think about your aging matters. As you'll recall from the first chapter, research shows that people who hold positive beliefs about aging live an average of seven and a half years longer than those who hold negative beliefs about aging. Further, those with positive age beliefs had significantly better physical and functional health over an eighteen-year period. With all the antiaging nonsense you encounter daily, it is critical not to slip back into negative beliefs. Revisit the grid below regularly to check in on your beliefs about aging.

JOYSPAN GRID	Your Thoughts About Growing Older
Expectations about aging	Growing older is improvement in some areas and decline in other areas.
Perspectives on control	The quality of my life is up to me.
Levels of effort	My efforts provide a path to an improved quality of life.
Reactions when obstacles arise	I persist in the face of challenge.
Relationships	I ask "How can I help you?"

In reviewing the grid, think about your expectations concerning aging and challenge any limiting beliefs about aging. Next, consider your perspective on control. Are you keeping in mind the things that you can control? Now, evaluate whether you are putting sufficient effort into your physical, mental, and emotional health in longevity. Remember to break goals into achievable steps. Instead of aiming to "get fit," commit to walking for fifteen minutes three times a week. Next, ask yourself, How am I viewing life's inevitable obstacles? Consider asking yourself, What's the next small step I can take? Finally, check in on your relationships. Are you making an effort to reach out to others? Are you more self-centered or others-centered? Where can you offer support?

Staying aware of your joyspan is a process of reflection, experimentation, and growth. By understanding the power of the butterfly effect, checking in with yourself daily, making small adjustments, and using the Joyspan Grid to guide your perspective, you can embrace life with greater joy and resilience. Over time, these small, intentional actions will ripple outward, transforming not just your own life, but also the lives of those around you.

JOYSPANNER: Oliver Sacks

The late Dr. Oliver Sacks, a neurologist, author, and scientist, was a towering figure in the fields of medicine and literature. Born on July 9, 1933, in London, Sacks combined his deep scientific expertise with a humanistic touch, bringing the lives of his patients to light in profound and inspiring ways.

> **GROW:** Dr. Sacks believed in lifelong learning and discovery. Even in his final years, he continued to write, publish, and explore the complexities of the human brain. In his memoir *On the Move: A Life* (2015), written at age eighty, he expressed his deep curiosity about the world. "I am still learning, still exploring," he wrote, "and I hope to be able to continue to do so until the very end."
>
> **CONNECT:** Dr. Sacks valued deep, meaningful connections with others, which were central to his joyspan. He described himself as an introvert and formed profound relationships with his patients, colleagues, and friends. His long-standing friendship with poet Thom Gunn and his correspondence with

countless readers of his books showed his ability to nurture relationships over decades.

ADAPT: Oliver Sacks was shy, closeted, and struggled with periods of professional isolation. His openness about his vulnerabilities and willingness to navigate the challenges in his life enabled him to adapt and thrive.

GIVE: Dr. Sacks's life was a testament to the power of giving. Through his books and essays, he gave voice to individuals whose stories might otherwise have gone unheard. His empathy and ability to find humanity in his patients inspired countless readers to think differently about illness, disability, and the human condition. Sacks gave generously of his time, mentoring younger neurologists, writers, and students. He frequently responded personally to the letters he received, offering encouragement, advice, and heartfelt thanks.

——— JOY PRACTICE: ———
Capitalize Upon What Gets Better as You Get Older

Strength	*Using It?*	*How?*
I don't care as much what others think of me.	☐ Yes ☐ No	
I have greater emotional stability.	☐ Yes ☐ No	
I draw upon experience-based problem-solving.	☐ Yes ☐ No	
I explore greater depth of spirituality.	☐ Yes ☐ No	
I choose to laugh.	☐ Yes ☐ No	

JOY PRACTICE:
How Is Your Joytank?

	When Your Joyspan Is High	Self-rating 1–10 1 = Strongly Disagree 2 = Disagree 3 = Neutral 4 = Agree 5 = Strongly Agree
Expectation About Aging	Growing older is improvement in some areas and decline in other areas.	
Perspective on Control	The quality of my life is up to me.	
Level of Effort	Effort provides a path to improved quality of life.	
Reaction When Obstacles Arise	Persist in the face of challenge.	
Relationships	I ask "How can I help you?"	

———— JOY PRACTICE: ————
Daily Check-In and Needed Tweaks

Check-In	Today I Feel	Helpful to Journal About It?	Need a Tweak? Here's a Starter List:	What I'll Try
How do I feel physically?	☐ Energetic ☐ Strong ☐ Tired ☐ Achy ☐ Something else	☐ Yes ☐ No	Take a ten-minute walk. Drink an extra glass of water each day. Stretch at home or in a yoga or stretch class. Have a nutritious snack.	
How do I feel mentally?	☐ Sharp ☐ Organized ☐ Foggy ☐ Something else	☐ Yes ☐ No	Increase your physical activity. Take steps to improve the quality and amount of your sleep. Check your medications and their side effects. Reduce or eliminate alcohol intake.	

(continued)

Check-In	Today I Feel	Helpful to Journal About It?	Need a Tweak? Here's a Starter List:	What I'll Try
How do I feel emotionally?	☐ Content ☐ Excited ☐ Stressed ☐ Sad ☐ Anxious ☐ Something else	☐ Yes ☐ No	Text, call, or write a letter, with no agenda, to someone—just to connect. Swap a passive activity (like watching TV) for something active, such as reading, painting, or gardening. Do a random act of kindness. Turn on some music and sing your heart out.	
Is there something in my day that will spark joy?	☐ Yes ☐ No	☐ Yes ☐ No	Create a list of things that bring you joy. Go outside in nature. Watch a comedy or read a funny book. Schedule time for a hobby that makes you lose track of time. Try something new—like cooking a new dish or visiting a new museum.	

CHAPTER 9

When Your Joyspan Dips

When a distracted driver slammed into the back of Ann's car on her sixty-second birthday, she was shaken but otherwise fine. The next morning, however, Ann had a sore neck and a pounding headache. Over the next few weeks, her headache didn't let up, she couldn't sleep, and she had to skip morning walks with friends and her Pilates classes.

Ann's husband was understanding at first, but when the headaches and sleeplessness didn't let up, she could tell he was bothered. Discouraged by not feeling well and deeply frustrated by the insomnia, Ann felt disconnected from her husband and friends and felt herself sinking. Everyday tasks felt heavy, housework piled up, and some days she never made it out of her pajamas. When their adult son came home for Thanksgiving, he noticed a change and asked if she was okay. She was quick to attribute her energy loss, messy home, and bedraggled appearance to getting old. "I'm absolutely fine," she explained. "It's just what happens with aging."

Only it isn't "just what happens with aging."

Too often, age is a scapegoat, taking the blame for negative circumstances. In this case, a car accident led to headaches, which led to sleep problems, which led to fatigue. Diminished physical health snowballed into feelings of disconnection, stagnation, and reduced self-worth. To Ann, it felt like the new normal of old age, a permanent reduction in the quality of her life.

It was not; it was a situational downward spiral of her emotional health, a temporary dip in her joyspan. The doctors diagnosed and provided treatment for her injury but even after her symptoms cleared she felt down and had to take action to re-chart her course.

When spirals threaten your joyspan, and they will, you need tools to stop the spin. Theodore Roosevelt said that comparison is the thief of joy. In working with people as they age, I regularly see five other thieves:

- Frustration: You feel discouraged by health problems and mobility limitations.
- Isolation: You feel left out or disconnected from friends or family.
- Burden: You feel like you are a nuisance.
- Loss: You feel heartbroken after losing a loved one.
- Defeat: You feel like the best days are all behind you.

Sometimes the thieves of joy arrive unnoticed. Other times they ambush you with great fanfare. It's not uncommon for the thieves to arrive together, frustration from a hip replacement coupled with the feeling of being a burden all wrapped in the wet blanket of feeling like your best days are behind you. When the thieves hijack you, joy feels like a companion who has wandered off, leaving you to navigate life's challenges alone. But joy isn't gone. Joy isn't a fragile, fleeting emotion. Joy resides within you, even when it's buried under layers of stress, grief, and disconnection. Like the sun, joy is always there. But when it's hidden by clouds, we mistakenly say it's gone. Joy is resilient and can break through the clouds because it is an innate part of the human experience.

It is important to recognize that joy and sorrow are *not* opposites; they often coexist. Allow yourself to feel both because when you grieve what's lost and embrace what remains, you create space for joy.

In this chapter we'll examine how to go about restoring emotional well-being when your joytank gets low.

THE SCIENCE BEHIND DIPS IN EMOTIONAL WELL-BEING

Slumps are part of the human experience, but they are not an inevitable consequence of aging. While physical health setbacks, social isolation, loss of loved ones, hopelessness, and internalized ageist beliefs can act as triggers, science shows that with intentional effort and the right strategies, you can rebound—and thrive—after emotional lows.

Emotional well-being is influenced by the interplay of biological, psychological, and social factors. Understanding the science behind these dips provides a road map for recovery.

You Feel Frustrated by Health Setbacks

Health problems can feel like an insurmountable drain of not only your physical energy but also your emotional resilience. Chronic pain, fatigue, or a sudden injury can disrupt the rhythm of your life, pulling you away from the activities and relationships that once brought meaning and joy. It's easy to sink into frustration or despair when these challenges seem to rob you of progress, leaving you feeling defeated. For Ann, what started as a minor car accident became a chain reaction: Aches turned into avoidance, and avoidance turned into isolation.

To move through a health setback, it helps to understand the connection between the body and the mind. Research consistently shows that physical activity can significantly improve mental health. Studies reveal that even light physical activity, such as walking for ten minutes, can reduce symptoms of depression by boosting endorphins and lowering stress hormones like cortisol. Practices like yoga and tai chi, which combine movement with mindfulness, offer relief not only for the body but also for the soul. These gentle forms of exercise are particularly accessible for those managing chronic pain or fatigue, making them a great starting point.

Another powerful tool is your mindset. Cognitive behavioral therapy (CBT) can help you reframe the discouraged thinking that accompanies health obstacles. CBT teaches you how to identify unhelpful thought patterns ("I'll never feel normal again") and replace them with more constructive ones ("Recovery is slow, but I'm taking steps forward"). When progress feels sluggish or nonexistent, this shift is transformative.

> "When we are no longer able to change a situation, we are challenged to change ourselves."
> —Viktor Frankl, psychiatrist and Holocaust survivor

Another crucial element of recovery is celebrating small victories. It can be tempting to compare yourself to your pre-setback self, but this often leads to discouragement. Instead, focus on incremental gains: getting a full night's sleep or walking a bit farther today than yesterday. Research on goal-setting emphasizes the power of breaking larger objectives into smaller, achievable steps. Each step not only brings you closer to physical recovery but also builds confidence and reinforces hope.

If persistent emotional challenges like anxiety or depression arise, a therapist can help you develop tailored strategies for coping. In addition, working with physiotherapists or rehabilitation specialists can ensure that your body's recovery is supported by expert guidance. Holistic approaches that combine physiotherapy, mental health counseling, and mindfulness-based practices like meditation have been shown to accelerate both physical and emotional healing.[1]

When health setbacks leave you feeling discouraged, don't underestimate the importance of community and connection. Loneliness worsens the psychological toll of a health setback, but leaning on trusted friends, family, or support groups can provide encouragement and perspective. Sharing your struggles with those who understand—or even those who are simply willing to listen—can make the journey feel less lonely. Research on social support highlights its role as a buffer against stress and a powerful predictor of recovery success.

Learning to navigate life with health problems is rarely a straight line—it's a winding road filled with highs and lows. But every effort you make toward coming to grips with it matters. The journey may feel long, but with persistence, self-compassion, and the right tools, recovery—and joy—are within reach.

You Feel Left Out or Disconnected

When you're not at your best, loneliness and isolation become a vicious cycle. It's natural to withdraw from others when you're feeling low, but withdrawal can deepen feelings of isolation, creating a feedback loop that's hard to escape. Research highlights the profound impact of loneliness on physical and mental health, equating its effects to smoking fifteen cigarettes a day and linking it to an increased risk of early mortality (see page 36). Still, reaching out can feel insurmountable when you're in the midst of a rough patch. How to begin?

Overcoming feelings of being left out begins with modest but intentional efforts to reconnect with others, even when it feels daunting.

Start by sharing how you're feeling with someone you trust. Vulnerability is often the bridge to deeper, more authentic relationships. Let a friend or family member know you're struggling, even if it's a simple message like "I've been feeling disconnected lately. Can we talk?" Vulnerability opens the door to connection. Being honest about your needs gives others the opportunity to show up for you.

For example, Ann felt invisible to her friends and separated from her family after her accident. Initially, she waited for others to notice her struggles and reach out—but they never did. Realizing she needed to take the first step, she started sending honest, vulnerable texts to a few close friends to let them know she was having a hard time. To her surprise, her openness was met with warmth and understanding. Encouraged, she joined a local book club, where discussing shared stories and laughing with strangers eventually turned into new friendships. Over time, these simple but intentional actions broke the cycle of isolation and reignited her sense of connection.

Try a group centered around your interests, as Ann did with her book club. Whether it's a fitness class, an a cappella group, or a film club, shared experiences provide opportunities to meet people who align with your passions. Participating in group activities fosters a sense of belonging and decreases feelings of loneliness. The impact is particularly strong when you shift your focus from yourself to meeting someone else's needs. Perhaps you teach at that film club, or drive someone to your fitness class. In doing this, you foster purpose and connection. Acts of kindness release oxytocin, the "bonding hormone," which can lift your mood and strengthen social ties.

Don't fall into the belief that others don't care about what you are going through or that your outreach will be met with rejection. These thoughts are often rooted in our insecurities rather than reality. Cognitive reframing—questioning whether your fears are based on facts or assumptions—can help you move forward with confidence.

Ann assumed that everyone thought she was making too much out of a small car accident, but it wasn't true. She pushed herself to reframe this thought into "Anyone who had such headaches and insomnia would struggle. People will understand." She replaced her initial thought with her chosen thought and reinforced it by writing about it each day. By reframing her thoughts, she rebuilt her sense of belonging.

You Feel Like a Burden

When your joytank plummets, you might feel that your struggles are a burden to those around you. This fear, though common, is often unfounded.[2] Close relationships thrive on mutual vulnerability. When you share your feelings with loved ones, you give them the opportunity to support you, deepening your connection rather than straining it.

When her son, noticing her withdrawal, asked if she was okay, Ann brushed off his concern. "I didn't want to worry him," she admitted later. "I thought I'd just deal with it on my own." But dealing with things on your own often leads to more isolation. When Ann opened up to her son about how she'd been feeling, he didn't see her as a burden. He saw her as someone he loved and wanted to help. When she finally did come clean, her bond with her son grew even stronger. Plus, she'd provided her son with a model of how to accept help.

To open channels of communication, share one specific feeling or challenge. For example, "I've been feeling really tired and down lately, and I'm not sure how to shake it." Be honest about your needs. If you need help, say so and be as specific as possible. Too often people want to help but don't know how. When a friend or family member asks how you are doing, expresses concern, or offers support, let them know their words matter to you.

My friend Kate, who was in a more serious car accident than Ann's, wasn't shy about making particular requests. She asked friends to take her shopping, meet her for short walks once a day, visit and just sit quietly while she rested, take her dog to the vet, and more. Not only did her friends feel relieved and grateful to know they were providing exactly what Kate wanted, but Kate recovered more quickly than her doctors expected—and she got her joy back sooner, too.

You might also consider joining a support group for your health issue, a book club, or a gentle, appropriate fitness class. Studies show that being part of a community improves emotional well-being, reduces feelings of loneliness, and even boosts physical health.[3] If you have mobility limitations, consider joining an online community. Virtual spaces can be as meaningful as in-person groups. Forums, Facebook groups, or apps like Meetup can connect you with others who share your interests or struggles.

Too often we put off joining a group until we feel better, but it is joining that helps us feel better. When Ann pushed herself to go to the first meeting of a volunteer group, she realized that everyone in the group was there for connection and support. That hour each month became a bright spot in her life, a reminder that she wasn't alone. Whether you're meeting new people or deepening existing relationships, connection is one of the most powerful tools for filling your joytank.

You Feel Heartbroken

When someone you love dies, it's not just the person you lose—it's the future you imagined with them, the shared routines, and the inside jokes. Research into grief emphasizes that "continuing bonds" with a loved one can help you cope. This doesn't mean clinging to the past but finding ways to maintain a sense of connection with the person you've lost. Write about the moments you cherished, the things you loved most about them, and the lessons they taught you. Studies show that expressive writing can help reduce the intensity of grief.[4] Consider putting together a **memory box** or creating a **small altar** of items that remind you of your loved one—photos, letters, or objects that hold significance. This can be a comforting way to revisit happy memories when you're ready.

When you're grieving, it's easy to feel like life has lost its meaning. But finding small moments of joy or purpose in your daily life can act as stepping stones toward healing. As difficult as it may feel, try writing down one thing each day that brought you comfort or peace, even if it's small—a warm cup of tea, the sound of birds outside your window, or a kind word from a friend. Art, music, or crafting can be outlets for processing emotions. Creative activities engage parts of the brain associated with healing. Don't pressure yourself to find "big" happiness. Instead, look for small moments—a beautiful sunset, a favorite meal, or a phone call with a friend. These moments can remind you that life still holds beauty, even in the midst of loss.

Grief can be isolating, especially if you feel like those around you don't understand the depth of your pain. But connecting with others who have experienced similar losses can be incredibly validating and healing. If you're religious or spiritual, seek comfort in rituals, prayers, or practices that align with your beliefs. Many people find solace in the idea of a continued connection with their loved one.

There will be moments when the grief feels unbearable—birthdays, anniversaries, or even random days when a smell, song, or place brings back a flood of memories. It's okay to cry, to scream, or to feel numb. Emotions are part of healing, and there's no "right" way to grieve. Call a friend or family member and let them know you're having a tough day. Even just saying, "I'm struggling today," can be a relief. On especially difficult days, plan activities that bring comfort—watching a favorite movie, going for a walk, or visiting a place that makes you feel close to your loved one.

You Feel Like the Best Days Are Behind You

When challenges start to mount, you may wonder if the best days are behind you. They don't have to be. Many people find their later years to be some of the most meaningful, productive, and joyful. Negative beliefs about aging, however, can act as a self-fulfilling prophecy. Individuals who hold negative stereotypes about aging are more likely to experience health issues, lower levels of happiness, and even shorter lifespans. Conversely, those who maintain a positive outlook on aging often live longer, healthier, and more fulfilling lives.

Ann, like many others, found herself stuck in a pattern of thinking that her low mood and energy were just an inevitable part of growing older. She caught herself labeling her struggles as permanent and viewing her life as one of inevitable decline. However, her perspective shifted when she decided to reframe her narrative. Instead of seeing her challenges as signs of decline, she began to view them as opportunities for growth. This reframing allowed her to find new purpose, and to rewrite her story in a way that celebrated resilience and possibility.

When we get stuck in negative thought patterns about aging, it's helpful to pause and reflect. Review the Joyspan Grid, which identifies common thought patterns when your joytank is running low.

	Low Joytank
Expectation about aging	Growing older means decline in every area of life.
Perspective on control	The quality of my life is out of my control.
Level of effort	Minimal; why bother when effort is fruitless?

Reaction when obstacles arise	Inclined to give up in the face of challenge.
Relationships	You place far more focus on "How can you help me?" rather than "How can I help you?"

When negative beliefs dominate, your expectations about aging might sound like this:

- "Growing older means inevitable decline in every area of life."
- "The quality of my life is out of my control."
- "Why bother trying? Nothing will change."
- "Challenges are too overwhelming; it's easier to give up."
- "Relationships only matter if people can help me."

These thoughts aren't just unhelpful—they're harmful. However, they can be challenged and replaced with more constructive, empowering beliefs. Here are steps you can take to turn your perspective around:

Find role models. Look for examples of older adults who have redefined what's possible in their later years. Let them inspire you to pursue your own goals, no matter your age. Stories of individuals who started businesses, learned new skills, or even completed physical feats like running marathons in their seventies or eighties can serve as powerful reminders that growth and adventure don't have an expiration date. Research shows that exposure to positive age beliefs and positive role models significantly influences our own beliefs and behaviors.[5]

Focus on possibilities rather than your limitations. It's natural to reminisce about the past, but fixating on what you've lost can block your view of what's still ahead. Instead, ask yourself: What do I want to learn, experience, or achieve in this chapter of my life? Whether it's mastering a new language, exploring a creative hobby, or deepening relationships with loved ones, focusing on future possibilities rather than past limitations can rekindle your sense of purpose. Positive psychology research emphasizes that goal-setting—even for small, achievable tasks—boosts both mental well-being and physical health.[6]

Take small, meaningful steps. Change doesn't have to be overwhelming. Start by setting manageable goals in the areas of life you'd like to improve. For example: If you feel disconnected from others, reach out to a friend or neighbor to grab coffee or join a local community group. If you're feeling stagnant, challenge yourself to learn something new—a skill, a recipe, or a craft. If you're doubting your physical abilities, start with gentle exercises like yoga or walking. Each small victory builds confidence and momentum.

Cultivate gratitude and self-compassion. Aging is not about avoiding challenges but rather embracing them with grace. Are you reflecting daily on what you're thankful for? Whether it's getting home safely from an outing, making a child laugh, or trying a particularly delicious new recipe, intentional daily gratitude improves emotional resilience and reduces stress.[7] Likewise, be kind to yourself. It's okay to have moments of doubt or low energy, but remind yourself that growth is possible at any age.

HOW ANN GOT HER JOY BACK

When her son came back into town for Easter, he noticed the change in his mother immediately. This time, she was interested in hearing all about his new job. There was a lightness in her voice that he hadn't heard in months.

If you're reading this because your joytank feels depleted, remember that it's not a permanent state. You have the power to rebuild, to reconnect, and to rediscover joy—even when it feels out of reach. It's not about fixing everything at once. It's about small steps. One walk. One conversation. One moment of gratitude.

> "When you come out of the storm, you won't be the same person who walked in. That's what the storm is all about."
> —*Haruki Murakami,* Kafka on the Shore

Ann was unaware of how dire her situation had become as she was living a muted version of her life on autopilot. The first step that Ann took was to recognize her empty joytank.

One cold December morning, Ann woke up and stared at the ceiling for an hour. She could hear Bill moving around downstairs, the clink of his coffee mug on the counter. Normally, the smell of freshly brewed coffee would be enough to pull her out of bed, but not today. When she finally dragged herself to the kitchen, Bill barely looked up from his newspaper. The air between them was thick with tension. Ann sat at the table, cradling her mug, and thought, *I can't keep living like this.* The thought startled her. For weeks, she had been drifting, feeling as though life was happening to her instead of something she was part of. But that morning, something shifted. She didn't know exactly what to do or where to start, but she decided that doing nothing wasn't an option anymore. Ann used the four essential elements of the Joyspan Matrix to rebuild her life. Through intentional efforts to grow, to connect, to adapt, and to give, Ann regained her joy.

Steps Toward Continued Growth

She started small. She opened her computer and typed in "chronic headaches." In one article, she read about post-concussion syndrome and was surprised to discover how common her symptoms were. This knowledge gave her a sense of relief: She wasn't broken or alone; she was healing. She took notes as she read, and it felt good to write. She started writing each evening, reflecting on her day and identifying something she was grateful for. Some days it was as simple as "the warmth of my blanket" or "the way the sunlight hit the snow." Over time, these reflections helped her shift her focus away from what she had lost and toward what she still had.

Rebuilding Connection

Isolation had subtly crept into Ann's life. She wasn't part of her vigorous walking group anymore, so she started to head out on her own. During these slow walks, she kept seeing the same older gentleman out walking his two golden retrievers. After seeing the trio a few times, she stopped to say hello and pet the dogs. They introduced themselves, and the next time she ran into Irving, he said, "Hello, Ann!" with such gusto that it made her laugh out loud. In their conversations, she learned that Irving was eighty-one and originally from Scotland. He told her how happy he was to get to walk his dogs every day on his "new knees." He'd had a double knee replacement four years before and was no longer in pain. The fact that he was out walking those big dogs inspired Ann and made her realize what was possible for her in her aging journey with the right mindset, patience, and effort.

She also made a point to reconnect with old friends who had made themselves scarce when she was down. She decided to put aside her hurt feelings by recognizing that they, too, had ups and downs in their lives. One evening, she texted a friend, explaining why she had disappeared and asking if she'd like to meet for coffee. The response was warm and encouraging, and Ann knew she was back on the right track.

Adapting to New Realities

One of the hardest lessons Ann had to learn was that she couldn't simply return to the way things were before the accident. Instead of fighting this reality, she embraced and adapted to it. She adjusted her schedule to allow for more rest, spreading out her tasks over several days instead of cramming them into one. She also experimented with new forms of exercise, like gentle yoga and tai chi, which felt less taxing on her body. Ann discovered that adapting didn't mean giving up; it meant finding new ways to thrive within her current circumstances.

Giving of Herself

While not feeling well physically and emotionally, Ann pulled away more and more from other people until her focus was entirely on herself. At her darkest, all her thoughts were on her own plight. She brainstormed ways to broaden her attention. She asked a neighbor who had four young children if she needed any help with carpooling the children. The mother was elated! She had to pick up two of the kids from different locations at 3:00 p.m. so it always required one to wait (resentfully) for nearly a half hour. Ann loved picking up the seven-year-old boy twice a week and she chuckled to herself as he'd talk the whole way home. He regaled her with detailed stories of playground battles over the rules of tetherball. "He grabbed the rope! You can't grab the rope, that's cheating, don't you think that's cheating?" The young mother was grateful for her help and had the children bring over lemons from their tree every week. Ann felt a sense of ease that she hadn't experienced in months. Giving her time and energy to help her harried neighbor reminded her that she could always choose to make a difference in the world (see figure 14).

FIGURE 14. Joyspan Matrix in Action: Ann, Age 86

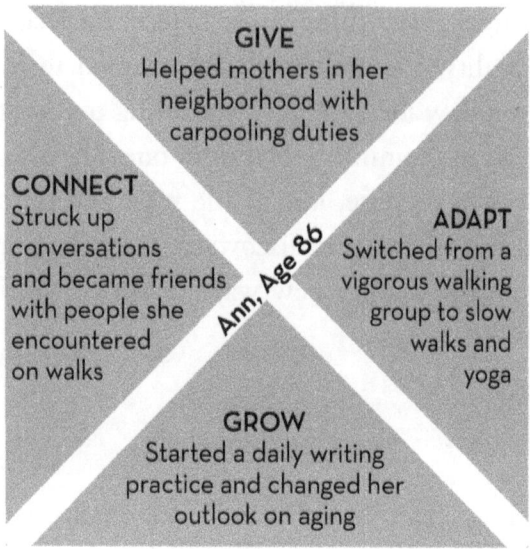

HOW TO FIND HELP

Asking for help feels especially daunting when you're already low. Yet, seeking help is one of the most powerful steps you can take toward restoring balance and finding joy again. Research consistently shows that reaching out for support, whether from professionals, loved ones, or community resources, is a key factor in overcoming emotional and physical challenges. When the world feels heavy, you don't have to navigate it alone. Help is out there, and asking for it is a sign of strength.

If you're feeling stuck or depleted, start by identifying how you feel. Are you feeling overwhelmed, isolated, or unsure of your next step? Journaling, speaking with a trusted friend, or simply sitting with your thoughts can help clarify your emotions. Self-awareness is a critical first step in problem-solving and emotional regulation. Give yourself permission to feel what you're feeling without judgment, as that is the foundation for taking action.

> "Anything that's human is mentionable, and anything that is mentionable can be more manageable."
> —Fred Rogers

Once you've identified how you are feeling, and what the dip might be about, reach out to someone. Share how you're feeling, even if it's as simple as saying, "I've been struggling a bit recently." Vulnerability deepens connections and paves the way for mutual support. Ann didn't want to share her struggles, fearing she'd burden others and seem incapable. Eventually, she mustered the courage to confide in a friend. With that nudge, Ann took small steps back to joy, gradually lifting her spirits and helping her rebuild her sense of purpose.

Try Professional Support

Therapy is one of the most effective tools for regaining balance and addressing emotional challenges. Therapists provide a safe, nonjudgmental space to explore your feelings and develop strategies for coping. Many communities offer sliding-scale or free counseling services. If you're unsure where to start, consider reaching out to your primary care doctor for recommendations or exploring online therapy platforms. If you need immediate support or don't know where to begin, helplines can provide guidance and connection to resources. In many countries, there are suicide and life crisis hotlines that offer 24-7 support for mental health crises. For nonemergencies, you can find specialized hotlines for grief, caregiving, or loneliness. Talking to a trained counselor, even briefly, can give you a real boost when your joyspan feels out of reach.

Rekindle Your Spiritual Life

Many people find solace in their spiritual practices, whether through prayer, meditation, or attending faith-based gatherings. Spirituality doesn't have to be tied to religion—it can also mean connecting with nature, practicing mindfulness, or reflecting on your values. Engaging in these practices can help you reconnect with a sense of purpose and hope, particularly during challenging times. There is a strong correlation between spiritual well-being and resilience.

When you feel depleted, it feels like you are the only one struggling. The truth is that millions of people face similar challenges, and there are resources, professionals, and communities ready to help. Take any step forward—no matter how tiny—to restore your joyspan: a cup of tea, a note to a friend, a warm bath, the quiet beauty of a sunrise—each moment of acknowledgment builds a bridge back to joy. When life is pulling you under, you can resurface. Joy, like light, has a way of finding its way back into even the darkest corners.

——— JOY PRACTICE: ———
When Your Joyspan Dips

What to Do	How to Do It	Write Your Response Here
Acknowledge the dip.	Start by naming what you're feeling—whether it's sadness, frustration, or fear—and recognize that it's valid.	
Share how you're feeling.	Share your feelings with someone you trust or a professional.	
Create a menu of possible steps.	If you are overwhelmed, break tasks into tiny pieces.	
Challenge your beliefs.	When thoughts like *Why bother?* arise, ask yourself: *Is this a fact or a feeling?* Remind yourself of times you've overcome challenges in the past.	
Practice gratitude... anyway.	Gratitude practices can increase happiness and reduce depressive symptoms. Keeping a gratitude journal or sharing three positive moments from your day with someone can be powerful.	

JOYSPANNER: Susie Forte

In 2017, Susie Forte's husband was killed in an ambush while on duty in Queensland, Australia. Feeling shocked and adrift, Susie decided that this tragedy would not be the end of their story.

> **GROW:** During the inquest into her husband's death, Susie decided to study law to advocate for others facing similar challenges. As a middle-aged woman who also had a full-time job to support her children, becoming a law student was a huge leap of personal transformation.
>
> **CONNECT:** The most important survival strategy Susie used for navigating the complexities of grief and rebuilding was staying in touch with her family, friends, and colleagues. She reached out to people even when she didn't feel like it, and she allowed herself to be honest about her pain and the emptiness and overwhelm she was experiencing.
>
> **ADAPT:** Transitioning in midlife to become a law student required significant adaptability. Susie managed the demands of her career, education, and family life, demonstrating flexibility in the face of adversity.
>
> **GIVE:** As a lawyer today, Susie advocates for domestic violence survivors. In addition to her paid work, she provides her services for a low fee or no cost for those who cannot afford to pay. Her commitment to giving back reflects a deep sense of purpose and dedication to making a positive impact in her community.

CONCLUSION

The Joyspan Legacy

The earliest seed of this book was planted when I was six years old, on a visit to my grandmother in a residential nursing facility. As the elevator doors opened on each floor, I glimpsed horrific scenes, from a hollow-cheeked man in a filthy sweatsuit slumped awkwardly in his wheelchair to a woman with white hair reaching toward me, moaning for assistance.

The suffering I saw stuck with me, and two decades later, I became a gerontologist. Have I improved older lives? I hope at least some. But not nearly enough. Real change and improvement come from those who are aging themselves. From you. It's never too late to make the internal and external changes that will impact your aging journey. The earlier you start, the better.

Having read this book, I believe you've put yourself on a positive path. You've replaced your fear of aging with confidence that you can handle whatever comes your way. Your feelings of helplessness have been replaced with knowing what you need to do today to fortify yourself for tomorrow. With this expanded understanding, you realize you are not destined to experience the same fate that your parents and grandparents possibly endured.

Your question is no longer how not to age, but how to age with vitality and purpose. You are not just after a long life. You want a long life in the best possible physical, mental, and emotional health. Your goal is not just to survive but to thrive, to intentionally maximize the quality of your life through the science of joyspan.

Joyspan, your well-being and satisfaction in longevity, is based on the science of psychological well-being. The four elements of the Joyspan Matrix are verbs, because action is required. You are on a lifelong journey in which you continue to:

- **Grow** by exploring, expanding, and trying new things.
- **Connect** by investing time and effort into new or existing relationships.
- **Adapt** by continually adjusting to new situations and conditions.
- **Give** by sharing of yourself.

I've had a front-row seat to the aging journeys of thousands of people. What I've seen has been both tragic and triumphant, horrifying and heartwarming. The problem isn't getting old or even dying. The problem is that for far too many people, the experience of getting older has been made unnecessarily painful and humiliating. We can change that. We are changing that. Joyspan matters because it reduces human suffering. By improving the quality of our long lives, we are paving the way for those who come after us, our children and our grandchildren and beyond.

When we take back our older lives and free ourselves from the fear-based, antiaging machine, we leave a legacy more valuable than any monetary inheritance. We show future generations that human dignity matters at every age and every stage.

I hope your long life is filled with growth, connection, adaptability, and giving. I hope you experience the joy of providing what society needs most now: wisdom, experience-based problem-solving, humility, spirituality, respect for art and nature, commitment to the greater good, and above all, love.

May your joyspan journey continue, knowing that aging is a privilege and that every day you live, you have the opportunity to create a joyful legacy. The work you do now echoes far beyond your lifespan. You are crafting not only your future but the future for generations to come. I wish you much joy in your travels.

Resources

BOOKS I LOVE

- *The Measure of Our Age* by M. T. Connolly
- *Being Mortal* by Atul Gawande
- *Breaking the Age Code* by Becca Levy
- *Elderhood* by Louise Aronson
- *The Book of Joy* by Dalai Lama and Desmond Tutu
- *The How of Happiness* by Sonja Lyubomirsky
- *Counting on Kindness* by Wendy Lustbader
- *The Let Them Theory* by Mel Robbins
- *Double Helix* by Robin Dellabough
- *Outlive* by Peter Attia
- *Learning to Speak Alzheimer's* by Joanne Koenig Coste
- *The Artist's Way* by Julia Cameron
- *The Comfort of Crows* by Margaret Renkl
- *Write a Must-Read* by AJ Harper
- *The Beautiful No and Other Tales of Trial, Transcendence, and Transformation* by Sheri Salata

INSTAGRAM ACCOUNTS I LOVE

- The_Gerontologist (It's mine... but I do love it)
- Aging Disgracefully
- SleepdocShelby
- IntegrativeClaire

- Endwellproject
- The_outdoor_therapist

PODCASTS I LOVE

- *Wiser Than Me* with Julia Louis-Dreyfus
- *Crow's Feet* with Melinda Blau
- *The Mel Robbins Podcast*
- *The Oprah Podcast*
- *The Drive* with Peter Attia
- *Huberman Lab*
- *The Practiced Life* with Sheri Salata
- *Good Life Project*
- *The Tony Robbins Podcast*
- *The Dr. Hyman Show*
- *Moonshots* with Peter Diamandis

Notes

INTRODUCTION

1. Louise Aronson, *Elderhood: Redefining Aging, Transforming Medicine, Reimagining Life* (Bloomsbury Publishing, 2019).

CHAPTER 1. What Is Joyspan?

1. Carol D. Ryff, "The Privilege of Well-Being in an Increasingly Unequal Society," *Current Directions in Psychological Science* 33, no. 5 (2024): 300–307.
2. A. Sutin et al., "Purpose in Life and Stress: An Individual-Participant Meta-Analysis of 16 Samples," *Journal of Affective Disorders* 345 (2024): 378–85.
3. Hod Orkibi, "Creative Adaptability: Conceptual Framework, Measurement, and Outcomes in Times of Crisis," *Frontiers in Psychology* 11 (2021): 588172.
4. Dalai Lama and Desmond Tutu, *The Book of Joy: Lasting Happiness in a Changing World* (Avery, 2016), 41.
5. *The Holy Bible, English Standard Version* (Crossway, 2001), Ps. 16:11.
6. R. Ito and A. Hayen, "Opposing Roles of Nucleus Accumbens Core and Shell Dopamine in the Modulation of Limbic Information Processing," *Journal of Neuroscience* 31, no. 16 (April 20, 2011): 6001–7.
7. Barbara L. Fredrickson and Thomas Joiner, "Reflections on Positive Emotions and Upward Spirals," *Perspectives on Psychological Science* 13, no. 2 (2018): 194–99.
8. Brené Brown, *Daring Greatly: How the Courage to Be Vulnerable Transforms the Way We Live, Love, Parent, and Lead* (Gotham Books, 2012).
9. A. Watts, *The Meaning of Happiness* (Harper & Row, 1940).
10. E. Dix et al., "Ageism in the Mental Health Setting," *Current Psychiatry Reports* 26 (2024): 583–90.
11. Becca R. Levy et al., "Age Beliefs and Physical Functioning: Longitudinal Findings from the Health and Retirement Study," *Journals of Gerontology* 79, no. 1 (2024): 123–32.

12. Nancy L. Pedersen et al., *Behavioral Genetics and Aging* (Oxford University Press, 2010).

CHAPTER 2. How Your Joyspan Affects Your Lifespan

1. Gina Kolata, "Live Long? Die Young? Answer Isn't Just in Genes," *New York Times*, August 31, 2006.
2. Pedersen et al., *Behavioral Genetics and Aging*.
3. Jeanne Calment (1875–1997) was a French supercentenarian who holds the record of the longest confirmed human lifespan, living to the age of 122 years and 164 days.
4. T. V. Pyrkov et al., "Longitudinal Analysis of Blood Markers Reveals Progressive Loss of Resilience and Predicts Human Lifespan Limit," *Nature Communications* 12, no. 1 (2021): 2765.
5. World Bank. (2024). *Life expectancy at birth, total (years)* [Data file]. Retrieved from https://data.worldbank.org/indicator/SP.DYN.LE00.IN.
6. M. A. Bernard (2024). Statement on the retirement of Dr. Marie Bernard. *National Institutes of Health*. Retrieved from https://www.nih.gov/about-nih/who-we-are/nih-director/statements/statement-retirement-dr-marie-bernard.
7. Saloni Dattani and Lucas Rodés-Guirao, "Why Do Women Live Longer Than Men?," *Our World in Data*, 2023.
8. Expert Market Research. (2024). *Anti-ageing market size, trends, growth & forecast to 2034*. Retrieved from https://www.expertmarketresearch.com/reports/anti-ageing-market.
9. David Snowdon, *Aging with Grace: What the Nun Study Teaches Us About Leading Longer, Healthier, and More Meaningful Lives* (Bantam, 2001).
10. Robert Waldinger and Marc Schulz, *The Good Life: Lessons from the World's Longest Scientific Study of Happiness* (Simon & Schuster, 2023).
11. Ed Diener and M. Y. Chan, "Happy People Live Longer: Subjective Well-Being Contributes to Health and Longevity," *Applied Psychology* 3, no. 1 (2011): 1–43.
12. J. Holt-Lunstad et al., "Social relationships and mortality risk: A meta-analytic review," *PLOS Medicine*, 7, no. 7 (2010): e1000316.
13. M. Blake, "Tackling a silent killer: Australia's loneliness epidemic," *The Australian*, November 22, 2024.
14. Z. Bian et al., "Genetic Predisposition, Modifiable Lifestyles, and Their Joint Effects on Human Lifespan: Evidence from Multiple Cohort Studies," *BMJ Evidence-Based Medicine* 29, no. 4 (2024): 255–63.
15. Bradley J. Willcox et al., "FOXO3: A Major Gene for Human Longevity," *Journals of Gerontology* 77, no. 8 (2022): 1479–88.

16. J. Lelieveld et al., "Effects of fossil fuel and total anthropogenic emission removal on public health and climate." *Proceedings of the National Academy of Sciences* 116, no. 15 (2019): 7192–97.
17. S. B. Rafnsson et al., "Loneliness, social integration, and incident dementia over 6 years: Prospective findings from the English Longitudinal Study of Ageing," *Journals of Gerontology: Series B* 75, no. 1 (2020): 114–24.
18. Becca Levy, *Breaking the Age Code: How Your Beliefs About Aging Determine How Long and Well You Live* (William Morrow, 2022).
19. Alan Rozanski et al., "Association of Optimism with Cardiovascular Events and All-Cause Mortality: A Systematic Review and Meta-Analysis," *JAMA Network Open* 2, no. 9 (2019): e1912200.
20. P. Jha et al., "21st-century hazards of smoking and benefits of cessation in the United States," *New England Journal of Medicine* 368, no. 4 (2013): 341–50.
21. A. Park, "The Man Who Thinks He Can Live Forever," *TIME*, September 20, 2023.

CHAPTER 3. How Your Joyspan Affects Your Healthspan

1. A. J. Cruz-Jentoft and A. A. Sayer, "Sarcopenia," *The Lancet,* 2019, 393(10191): 2636–46.
2. Centers for Disease Control and Prevention, "How Much Physical Activity Do Older Adults Need?," last modified October 7, 2022.
3. Douglas Paddon-Jones et al., "Protein and Healthy Aging," *American Journal of Clinical Nutrition* 99, no. 6 (2014): 1243S–48S.
4. P. Verhaeghen, "Aging and Vocabulary Score: A Meta-Analysis," *Psychology and Aging* 18, no. 2 (2003): 332–39.
5. I. Grossman et al., "Reasoning About Social Conflicts Improves into Old Age," *Proceedings of the National Academy of Sciences* 107, no. 16 (2010): 7246–50.
6. Alzheimer's Disease International, "Numbers of People with Dementia Worldwide," last modified November 30, 2020, https://www.alzint.org.
7. World Health Organization, "Global Action Plan on the Public Health Response to Dementia" 2017–2025, March 15, 2023.
8. Bruce S. McEwen and John H. Morrison, "The Brain on Stress: Vulnerability and Plasticity of the Prefrontal Cortex Over the Life Course," *Neuron* 79, no. 1 (2013): 16–29.
9. World Health Organization. (2024). *Mental health.* https://www.who.int/health-topics/mental-health.
10. Erin Trifilio et al., "Changes in Emotions and Mood with Aging," in *Cognitive Changes and the Aging Brain*, ed. Kenneth M. Heilman and Stephen E. Nadeau (Cambridge University Press, 2019), 127–39.

11. J. Jurgaitis et al., "Changes in cognition, depression and quality of life after carotid revascularisation: A prospective study," *Journal of Clinical Medicine* 8, no. 8 (2019): 1136.
12. G. E. Vaillant, *Triumphs of Experience: The Men of the Harvard Grant Study* (Belknap Press of Harvard University Press, 2012).
13. C. S. Carver and M. F. Scheier, "Dispositional Optimism," *Trends in Cognitive Sciences* 18, no. 6 (2014): 293–99, doi: 10.1016/j.tics.2014.02.003, PMID: 24630971; PMCID: PMC4061570.

CHAPTER 4. Grow with Joy

1. S. Papert, *Mindstorms: Children, Computers, and Powerful Ideas* (Basic Books, 1980).
2. Carol D. Ryff, "Psychological Well-Being Revisited: Advances in the Science and Practice of Eudaimonia," *Psychotherapy and Psychosomatics* 83, no. 1 (2013): 1028.
3. Susan T. Charles, "Mental Well-Being and Lifelong Learning," *Journals of Gerontology: Series B* 75, no. 3 (2020): 557–67.
4. Carl R. Rogers, *On Becoming a Person: A Therapist's View of Psychotherapy* (Houghton Mifflin, 1961), 17.
5. Kristin D. Neff, *Self-Compassion: The Proven Power of Being Kind to Yourself* (HarperCollins, 2011), 22.
6. "Accepting Yourself as You Are: Practicing the Sixth Mantra," Thich Nhất Hạnh, lecture at Lower Hamlet, Plum Village, January 15, 2012.
7. David Steindl-Rast, *Gratefulness, the Heart of Prayer: An Approach to Life in Fullness* (Paulist Press, 1984), 25.
8. Richard B. Nussbaum et al., "Gratitude, Subjective Well-Being, and Self-Acceptance in Older Adults: The Role of Daily Journaling," *Aging & Mental Health* 25, no. 6 (2021): 933.
9. Brené Brown, *Daring Greatly: How the Courage to Be Vulnerable Transforms the Way We Live, Love, Parent, and Lead* (Gotham, 2012), 34.
10. Paul J. Silvia and Christopher R. Berg, "Curiosity and Resilience in Older Adults," *Aging and Mental Health* 18, no. 6 (2012): 745–53.
11. Frederick W. Unverzagt et al., "Effects of Memory Training on Cognitive Function in Older Adults: Results from the ACTIVE Study," *Journal of the American Geriatrics Society* 55, no. 2 (2007): 294–301.
12. G. Livingston et al., "Dementia prevention, intervention, and care," *The Lancet* 390(10113) (2017): 2673–734.

13. Susan Krauss Whitbourne, "How to Keep Your Brain Sharp as You Age," *Psychology Today*, last modified February 20, 2020, https://www.psychologytoday.com/us/blog/fulfillment-any-age/202002/how-keep-your-brain-sharp-you-age.
14. Paul B. Baltes and Margret M. Baltes, "Psychological Perspectives on Successful Aging: The Model of Selective Optimization with Compensation," in *Successful Aging: Perspectives from the Behavioral Sciences*, ed. Paul B. Baltes and Margret M. Baltes (Cambridge University Press, 1990), 1–34.
15. Elizabeth W. Dunn, "Curiosity, Empathy, and the Social World," *Journal of Social and Personal Relationships* 32, no. 7 (2015): 789–804.
16. J. Aaker and N. Bagdonas, *Humor, Seriously: Why Humor Is a Secret Weapon in Business and Life* (Crown, 2021).
17. Michael Miller et al., "The Impact of Laughter on Cardiovascular Health," *American Journal of Cardiology* 90, no. 3 (2022): 231–39.
18. Lee Berk et al., "Humor, Cortisol Reduction, and Cognitive Flexibility in Older Adults," *Journal of Psychosomatic Research* 128 (2021): 43–49.
19. Sarah Crawford and Marie Caltabiano, "Humor as a Coping Mechanism for Psychological Distress in Older Adults: Benefits and Limitations," *Journal of Mental Health and Aging* 6, no. 3 (2020): 145–61.
20. Dalai Lama and Desmond Tutu, *The Book of Joy: Lasting Happiness in a Changing World* (Avery, 2016).
21. Anthony Ong, "The Role of Humor and Laughter in Health and Well-Being," *Psychology and Aging* 26, no. 1 (2011): 158–66.

CHAPTER 5. Connect to Joy

1. Julianne Holt-Lunstad, "The Potential Public Health Relevance of Social Isolation and Loneliness: Prevalence, Epidemiology, and Risk Factors," *Public Policy & Aging Report* 27, no. 4 (2017): 127–30.
2. American Psychiatric Association, "New APA Poll: One in Three Americans Feels Lonely Every Week," January 30, 2024.
3. Daniel W. Russell, "UCLA Loneliness Scale (Version 3): Reliability, Validity, and Factor Structure," *Journal of Personality Assessment* 66, no. 1 (1996): 20–40.
4. Robin Dunbar, *Friends: Understanding the Power of Our Most Important Relationships* (Little, Brown, 2021).
5. V. Kaufman et al., "Unique Ways in Which the Quality of Friendships Matter for Life Satisfaction," *Journal of Happiness Studies* 23 (2022): 2563–80.
6. Laura L. Carstensen, "The Influence of a Sense of Time on Human Development," *Science* 312, no. 5782 (2006): 1913–15.

7. William J. Chopik, "The Benefits of Knowing People Across the Life Span," *Social Psychological and Personality Science* 8, no. 1 (2017): 37–44.
8. Stephen R. Covey, *The 7 Habits of Highly Effective People: Powerful Lessons in Personal Change* (Free Press, 1989).
9. Julianne Holt-Lunstad, (2017): 127–30.
10. Tina J. Klinkenberg et al., "Family Communication and Satisfaction in the Elderly," *Journal of Family Psychology* 34, no. 2 (2020): 158–68.

CHAPTER 6. Adapt with Joy

1. Information Now, Grandparent Issues, https://www.informationnow.org.uk/article/grandparent-issues/
2. Centre for Better Ageing, 'Retirement Transitions in Later Life', 5 October 2017, https://ageing-better.org.uk/news/retirement-transitions-later-life
3. T. Saito and I. Kai, "What Factors Affect the Evolution of the Wife's Mental Health After the Husband's Retirement? A Longitudinal Analysis in Japan," *Journal of Epidemiology* 31(4): 234–41.
4. Office for National Statistics, 'Profile of the Older Population Living in England and Wales in 2021 and Changes Since 2011', 3 April 2023, https://www.ons.gov.uk/peoplepopulationandcommunity/birthsdeathsandmarriages/ageing/articles/profileoftheolderpopulationlivinginenglandandwalesin2021andchangessince2011/2023-04-03
5. George A. Bonanno, *The Other Side of Sadness: What the New Science of Bereavement Tells Us About Life After Loss* (Basic Books, 2009).
6. Richard G. Tedeschi and Lawrence G. Calhoun, "The Posttraumatic Growth Inventory: Measuring the Positive Legacy of Trauma," *Journal of Traumatic Stress* 9, no. 3 (1996): 455–71.

CHAPTER 7. Give with Joy

1. Stephen Post and Jill Neimark, *Why Good Things Happen to Good People: How to Live a Longer, Happier, Healthier Life by the Simple Act of Giving* (Broadway Books, 2007).
2. Daryl R. Van Tongeren et al., "Prosociality Enhances Meaning in Life," *Journal of Positive Psychology* 11, no. 3 (2016): 225–36.
3. Will Stor, "A Better Happiness," *New Yorker*, July 7, 2016.
4. Barbara L. Fredrickson et al., "A Functional Genomic Perspective on Human Well-Being," *Proceedings of the National Academy of Sciences* 110, no. 33 (2013): 13684–89.
5. Brian R. Little, *Personal Project Pursuit: Goals, Action, and Human Flourishing* (Lawrence Erlbaum Associates, 2007).

6. Elizabeth W. Dunn et al., "Spending Money on Others Promotes Happiness," *Science* 319, no. 5870 (2008): 1687–88.
7. UCLA Bedari Kindness Institute, "Observing Acts of Kindness Inspires Prosocial Behavior," 2022, newsroom.ucla.edu.
8. A. Kumar and N. Epley, *University of Texas at Austin Study: Underestimating the Impact of Kindness*, 2022, studyfinds.org.
9. P. L. Hill et al., "Collegiate Purpose Orientations and Well-Being in Early and Middle Adulthood," *Journal of Applied Developmental Psychology* (2009), doi:10.1016/j.appdev.2009.12.001.
10. *The Bible, New King James Version*, Ps. 46:10

CHAPTER 8. Filling Your Joytank

1. Vithya Velaithan et al., "The Association of Self-Perception of Aging and Quality of Life in Older Adults: A Systematic Review," *Gerontologist* 64, no. 4 (April 2024).
2. K. M. Sheldon et al., "The Independent Effects of Goal Contents and Motives on Well-Being: It's Both What You Pursue and Why You Pursue It," *Personality and Social Psychology Bulletin* 30, no. 4 (2004): 475–86.
3. L. L. Carstensen et al., "Emotional Experience Improves with Age: Evidence Based on Over Ten Years of Experience Sampling," *Psychology and Aging* 26, no. 1 (2011): 21.
4. Z. Zimmer et al., "Spirituality, Religiosity, Aging and Health in Global Perspective: A Review," *SSM Population Health* 2 (2016): 373–81.
5. H. G. Koenig et al., *Handbook of Religion and Health*, 2nd ed. (Oxford University Press, 2012).
6. D. R. Hodge and S. Burchfield, "Spirituality, Religiosity, and Mortality: Examining the Relationship in Older Adults," *Aging Clinical and Experimental Research*, 2023.
7. Pope Francis, "The Gifts of Aging," 2023.
8. Jane Kuepfer, "'God Just Isn't Finished with Me Yet': Meaning, Memory and Mystery Are Part of the Aging Process," *Canadian Mennonite*, June 18, 2018.
9. Edward N. Lorenz, *The Essence of Chaos* (University of Washington Press, 1993).

CHAPTER 9. When Your Joyspan Dips

1. J. Kabat-Zinn, *Full Catastrophe Living: Using the Wisdom of Your Body and Mind to Face Stress, Pain, and Illness* (Delacorte, 1990).
2. S. Levine et al., "The Role of Mutual Vulnerability," *Social Cognitive and Affective Neuroscience* (2015).
3. J. Holt-Lunstad et al., "Loneliness and Health," *PLoS Medicine* (2010).

4. R. A. Neimeyer and D. C. Sands, "Expressive Writing Changes Grief into Meaning: Toward a Model of Meaning Reconstruction in Bereavement," *Death Studies* 35, no. 6 (2011): 535–58.
5. B. R. Levy et al., "Association Between Positive Age Stereotypes and Recovery from Disability in Older Persons," *JAMA* 308, no. 19: 1972–73.
6. J. A. Cook et al., "Whole Health Action Management: A Randomized Controlled Trial of a Peer-Led Health Promotion Intervention," *Psychiatric Services* 71, no. 3 (2020): 246–54.
7. D. R. Cregg and J. S. Cheavens, "Gratitude Interventions: Effective Self-Help? A Meta-Analysis of the Impact on Symptoms of Depression and Anxiety," *Journal of Happiness Studies* 22, no. 1 (2021): 413–45.

Acknowledgments

Todd Burnight, my best friend and husband of thirty years, you've been constantly encouraging and incredibly kind. I can never thank you enough for your steadfast goodness and all the laughs. Our children, Beau, Claire, and Elle, believed in my ability to write a book and that made me believe it, too. I adore and admire each of you for your goodness and commitment to your unique missions in life. Savor every day of it.

My mom, Betty, is my daily delight and my inspiration. You provide an example of what a long joyspan looks like and the work it takes to achieve it. My dad, John Parker, encouraged me from heaven and sat with me during the long hours of writing. With my dad and God, I was never alone.

Jennifer Thompson, my agent, you are a dream in every way, wise, hilarious, encouraging, and someone I admire so much. Jenny Baumgartner, Daisy Blackwell Hutton, and Beth Adams, my outstanding editors at Hachette, you purchased this book for Hachette and your expertise and faith made it so much better. The brilliant Danielle Claro brought Robin Dellabough into my life and changed my life forever. Robin, your vision, integrity, expertise, and no-nonsense editing completely transformed this book. Thank you.

My siblings, KC, Russ, and Karen, you inspire me by your aging journeys and I love you so very much. Our sweet family is everything to us and thank you, Paige, Courtney, Jimmy, Katie, Stephen, Parker,

Manu, Marshall, Dessie, Lee, Lauren, Shane, Andy, Maggie, Greg, Shannon, Carol, Larry, Cole, Hayden, Nash, Rusty, Belinda, John Parker, Mack, Tait, Maddy, Finya, Kasper, Ford, Charley, Kaia, and Florence. Cherished forever friends, Elise Fields, Marina Glava, Lisa Ayotte, Ira Ehrenpreis, Colleen Premer, Andrea Martin, Liz Gately, Mary Tips, Courtnay November, Laura Mosqueda. MT Connelly, Liz Zelinski, Kate Wilber, Sherry Zamanigan, Angie Haskins, Joanna Mann, Meredith Miller, Cary Wallin, Kathy Mundy, Margo Ludwig, Shana Hill, Abbas Zahawi, Kathy Purdy, Mary Tips, Mercedes Wagner, AJ Harper, Laura Stone, Kimmy Darling, Kerry Wagner, Jan Carson and the Aging Brilliantly founders group, and my first friend, Annie Mortensen.

Last but not least, my best girlfriend and soulmate, Cindy McCormick, you were there every day of the long writing process and the daily onslaught of ideas and Peleton-induced titles.

About the Author

Dr. Kerry Burnight is on a mission to make older better. She taught geriatric medicine and gerontology for eighteen years at the University of California, Irvine, School of Medicine. She is the cofounder of the nation's first Elder Abuse Forensic Center and founder of TheGerontologist.com. She was an invited speaker to the White House at the Elder Justice Summit, and at the U.S. Department of Justice. She has appeared on *CBS News*, *NBC News*, *The Doctors*, *Money Matters*, and *Dr. Phil* and has been the keynote speaker at hundreds of conferences. She's known as "America's Gerontologist" for optimizing dignity, health, and joy in longevity through her research, teaching, podcasts, blogs, Instagram, X, Facebook, and TikTok.